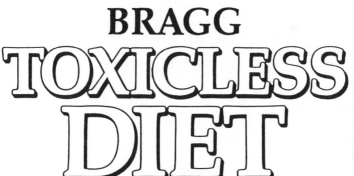

BRAGG
TOXICLESS DIET

BODY PURIFICATION & HEALING SYSTEM

THE DIET THAT CAN KEEP YOU AGELESS!

Proven & Used by Millions World-Wide
For a Youthful, Painfree, Tireless Body &
Physical, Mental & Spiritual Rejuvenation!

By
PAUL C. BRAGG, N.D., Ph.D.
LIFE EXTENSION SPECIALIST
and
PATRICIA BRAGG, N.D., Ph.D.
LIFE EXTENSION NUTRITIONIST

HEALTH SCIENCE
Box 7, Santa Barbara, California 93102 U.S.A.

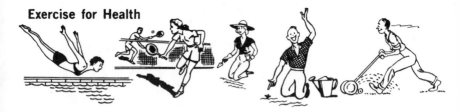
Exercise for Health

TOTAL HEALTH FOR THE TOTAL PERSON

In a broad sense, "Total Health for the Total Person" is a combination of physical, mental, emotional, social, and spiritual components. The ability of the individual to function effectively in his environment depends on how smoothly these components function as a whole. Of all the qualities that comprise an integrated personality, a well-developed, totally fit body is one of the most desirable.

A person may be said to be totally physically fit if they function as a total personality with efficiency and without pain or discomfort of any kind. That is to have a Painless, Tireless, Ageless body, possessing sufficient muscular strength and endurance to maintain an effective posture, successfully carries on the duties imposed by the environment, meets emergencies satisfactorily and has enough energy for recreation and social obligations after the "work day" has ended, meets the requirements for his environment through efficient functioning of his sense organs, possesses the resilience to recover rapidly from fatigue, tension, stress and strain without the aid of stimulants, and enjoys natural sleep at night and feels fit and alert in the morning for the job ahead.

Keeping the body totally fit and functional is no job for the uninformed or the careless person. It requires an understanding of the body, sound health and eating practices, and disciplined living. The results of such a regimen can be measured in happiness, radiant health, agelessness, peace of mind, in the joy of living and high achievement.

Paul C. Bragg and Patricia Bragg

Dear friend, I wish above all things that thou may prosper and be in health even as the soul prosper—3 John:2

JOIN

The Bragg Crusades for a 100% Healthy, Vigorous, Strong America and a Better World for All!

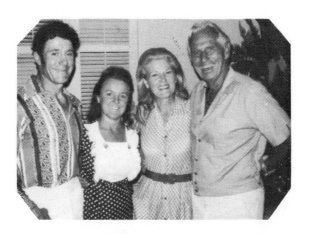

Jack LaLanne, Patricia Bragg, Elaine LaLanne & Paul Bragg

Jack says, "Bragg saved my life at age 14 when I attended the Bragg Crusades in Oakland, California." From that day on Jack has lived the health life and teaches Health & Fitness to millions.

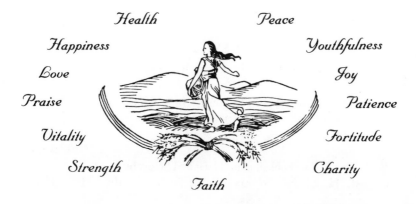

Health   Peace

Happiness   Youthfulness

Love   Joy

Praise   Patience

Vitality   Fortitude

Strength   Charity

Faith

BRAGG
TOXICLESS
DIET

BODY PURIFICATION
& HEALING SYSTEM

By
PAUL C. BRAGG, N.D., Ph.D.
LIFE EXTENSION SPECIALIST
and
PATRICIA BRAGG, N.D., Ph.D.
LIFE EXTENSION NUTRITIONIST

- REVISED -
Copyright © Health Science

Twenty-sixth printing MCMXCII
ISBN: 0-87790-033-7

Published in the United States by
HEALTH SCIENCE - Box 7, Santa Barbara, Calif. 93102, USA

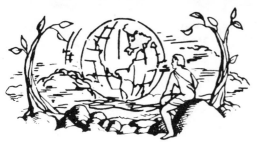

CONTENTS

"To preserve health is a moral and religious duty, for health is the basis for all social virtues. We can no longer be useful when not well."

— Dr. Samuel Johnson, Father of Dictionaries

◇◇◇

continued over page

Contents

Our Favorite Quotes We Share With You
(you will find them where space allows)

---

*The book that will benefit most is the one that inspires men
to think and to act for themselves. —Elbert Hubbard*

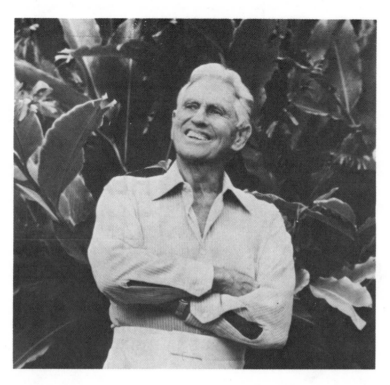

PAUL C. BRAGG, N.D., Ph.D.

Life Extension Specialist, World Health Crusader, Pioneer Nutritionist, one of the world's foremost authorities on scientific nutrition and physical fitness, at his home in Hawaii.

JOIN THE FUN AT THE "BRAGG LONGER LIFE, HEALTH AND HAPPINESS CLUB" WHEN IN HAWAII

Be sure to visit the "Longer Life, Health and Happiness Club" at Fort DeRussy, right at Waikiki Beach, Honolulu, Hawaii. Membership is free and open to everyone who wishes to attend any morning Monday through Saturday from 9:00 to 10:30 a.m. for deep breathing, exercising, meditation, group singing and mini-health lectures on how to live a long, healthy life! The group averages 75 to 100 per day. When Paul and Patricia Bragg are away lecturing, they have their leaders carry on until their return. Thousands have visited the club from around the world and then they carry the message of health and happiness to their friends and relatives back home. Paul and Patricia extend an invitation to you and your friends to join the club for health and happiness fellowship with them . . . when you visit Hawaii!

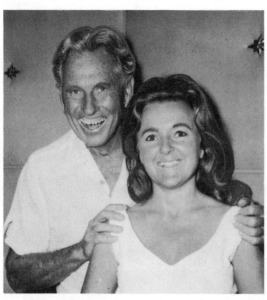

LIFE'S GREATEST TREASURE IS RADIANT HEALTH

Paul C. Bragg and daughter Patricia say, "There is no substitute for Health. Those who possess it are richer than kings."

KEEP YOUNG BIOLOGICALLY WITH EXERCISE AND GOOD NUTRITION

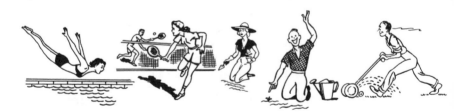

You can always remember that you have the following good reason for sticking to your health program:

- The ironclad laws of Nature.
- Your common sense which tells you that you are doing right.
- Your aim to make your health better and your life longer.
- Your resolve to prevent illness so that you may enjoy life.
- By making an art of life, you will be young at any age.
- You will retain your faculties and be hale, hearty, active and useful far beyond the ordinary length of days, and you will also possess superior mental and physical powers.

THE TOXICLESS DIET BODY PURIFICATION AND HEALING SYSTEM

The Natural and Scientific Plan
of Eating and Fasting
Your Way to Super Health

A COMPLETE Course of Instructions for those who desire to learn How to Control their Health and Prolong their Life.

By starting this New Way of Living you can gain its wonder-working benefits in every area of life within two short weeks.

See for yourself that every page is crammed full of practical, down-to-earth, easy-to-understand knowledge that you can put to work for you right on the spot. See for yourself that here at last is a Health System that WORKS!

This startling book helps you find and draw upon your body's natural sources of Vitality, Energy, and Vigour. It teaches you to free yourself of the health wreckers that are tearing your body apart. It will teach you how to flush the toxic poisons out of your body, that cause most of your body miseries. It helps eliminate stress, strain, tensions and fatigue. It helps you find sparkling new supplies of zest and energy ready when you need them. If tensions, stresses and strains are depleting your vitality supplies—if fatigue and exhaustion are robbing you of energy—here is the Golden Key to a Fresh, New Adventure in Living. How to stay youthful and active until you are 100. It's designed to give you the look of a youthful person even when past sixty; to keep you sexually active and vital beyond your seventies, and in radiant good health until 100 or more. Here is one of the most natural, simplest and gentlest, and yet truly revolutionary, anti-ageing, anti-misery plans ever invented by the mind of man.

THE TOXICLESS DIET BODY PURIFICATION AND HEALING SYSTEM FULLY EXPLAINED

First, I want it definitely understood that this System is not one that claims to cure disease.

No System can " cure " disease. No person can " cure " you of your ailments, aches, pains and diseases. Only the internal functions of your own body banishes diseases. The human body is self-repairing and self-healing. You break a bone, the doctor sets the bone and puts it into a cast. The broken bone knits together again; after a certain number of weeks the bone is again as strong as it was before the break. The internal healing forces that are within every human body, healed and renewed the bone. There is no special diet, no special food, no pill, no injection or prescription that can " cure " or mend a broken bone.

Only NATURE CURES. Burn that into your consciousness. Only NATURE CURES.

Every human body has a special built-in healing mechanism. You cut your hand, three to five stitches are required to close up the open wound, the doctor stitches the wound, he cleans the wound, he bandages the wound and then he can do no more. Now the healing mechanism of your body starts the work of healing.

YOUR BODY'S VITAL FORCE

To simplify this explanation of the Toxicless Diet Body Purification and Healing System I am going to call this healing power—Vital Force.

All of us must have Vital Force in order to stay alive. When the Vital Force is completely exhausted, then there is death.

We must have Vital Force in order to stay alive. It is true that many people live in a very low rate of physical vibration because they have a very low rate of Vital Force. Then there are people who live by a daily health programme who enjoy a high rate of physical vibration; their Vital Force is high.

Every day of your life you meet people with a high amount of Vital Force. On the other hand, every day you see tired, exhausted, nervous, frustrated people full of aches, pains, disease, stresses, strains and tensions. Most of these people are prematurely old . . . that is they are older than their calendar years.

People with a low quota of Vital Force have a low resistance to infectious diseases . . . they are the people who have frequent colds, flu, strep throat and many, many other infectious diseases.

8

They are the people who are chronically fatigued. They are the people with poor memories. They are the people who are full of aches and pains. They are the people who are pale and blood-less. They are the unhappy people. They are the irritable people.

LACK OF VITAL FORCE BRINGS ON ENERVATION

With the Vital Force at a low ebb enervation takes over. And when enervation takes over physical troubles start to multiply.

Remember first and foremost that we are instruments. In order for this fine instrument called the human body to operate efficiently there must be an adequate amount of Vital Force to keep the eliminative organs removing the poisons from our bodies.

There you have the secret of life in a nut-shell. The body builds a certain amount of toxic poison from the food you eat. As the food passes through the gastro-intestinal tract, the great intelligence of the body selects the nutrients it needs, and the waste or residue is passed on and out of the body. This function requires a large amount of Vital Force. If a person has a low amount of Vital Force the food wastes do not pass out of the body in the required time.

The body has a high temperature of 98.6 and if food wastes remain too long in the hot gastro-intestinal tract toxic poisons build up, auto-intoxication and putrefaction starts to set in. This toxic poison is then thrown back into the blood stream, thus you start to poison yourself! What is the effect of this toxic poison being thrown back into the main blood stream?

Nature always gives warnings when toxic poisons start to build up in the bloodstream. There are headaches, headaches of all degrees, some that ache, others that throb and then the worst of all, the deadly migraine headache.

There are many other symptoms of auto-intoxication—biliousness, nausea, mental depression, irritability, stresses, tensions and strains. The full list of symptoms is far too long to list here.

So we see that enervation slows down the eliminative functions, not only of the bowels but also the kidneys, skin and lungs. They just cannot eliminate the toxic poisons from the body when the Vital Force is low.

CAUSE AND EFFECT

For every effect there must be a cause. All these pathological (Disease) conditions are effects of a common cause . . . enervation.

The basic cause of enervation is, of course, poor diet. The average food of civilization has been so perverted and robbed of virgin nature that most of its vital substances have been removed. You cannot expect to build a high Vital Force on poor fuel. Most humans in civilization suffer from chronic malnutrition. The word "mal" means faulty. So malnutrition means faulty nutrition.

Twenty-five hundred years ago on the Island of Cos, in classical Greece, a bearded physician-teacher, Hippocrates, sat in the shade of an Oriental plane tree on a beautiful hillside and admonished his bright-eyed circle of medical students in one of his most pithy and precise aphorisms: *"THY FOOD WILL BE YOUR REMEDY"*. NO ONE, TO DATE, HAS MORE ELOQUENTLY GIVEN US A WAY OF LIFE.

The entire Toxicless Diet Body Purification and Healing System is based on this one great thought . . .

"THY FOOD WILL BE YOUR REMEDY"

This System is based on the idea that in the correct food (Natural Food) MAN CAN PURIFY HIS BODY AND FIND PERFECT HEALTH AGAIN.

I believe and I have proved over the last seventy-five years that within fruits and vegetables are the natural remedies for all of man's physical problems.

The healing profession insists it strives to emulate the Father of all physicians and, indeed, is required before licensing, to take the Hippocratic Oath, one of the most sublime declamations for lofty ethical standards ever written. Yet today there are thousands of dedicated bacteriologists, pharmaceutical researchers and chemists sitting in gleaming white laboratories in every major city throughout the world, busily turning out synthetic, magic panaceas for every human misery. Unlike that of the venerable Hippocrates, their battle cry appears to be: "Thy remedy shall be our newly invented wonder remedy".

Look at your T.V. commercials . . . one after the other, the old and new remedies flash on the screen. We have all heard "Fast, fast relief for headaches with this remedy or the other". "Fast, fast relief for acid stomach, heart-burn and indigestion. If your joints and muscles hurt . . . take this fast, fast remedy".

Not only the T.V., but also the radio, the newspapers and magazines are full of remedies for all kinds of human ailments.

Unhappily, anxiety-ridden people, following the warning voices of televised drug commercials and newspaper advertisements, consider health and energy something that they can purchase in a bottle—powder or pill form at the chemist drug shop; they forget

10

or never knew, that health can be found only by obeying the clear-cut laws of Nature.

The Toxicless Diet Body Purification and Healing System is the intelligent following of the clear-cut laws of Nature.

People today with ailments are constantly looking for a " Cure-all ". They are looking for the miracle substance which will restore them back to Health and Youth.

FOOD CAN MAKE OR BREAK YOU

People are so steeped in their rotten habits of eating that they think there is some mysterious potion that will benefit all of their physical miseries. They want to circumvent all their bad habits of eating. They will not get it into their thick skulls that food can make you a physical wreck; or, it can give you Health Supreme!

DIRTY BLOOD IS THE CAUSE OF ILLNESS AND PREMATURE AGEING

Humans will not face the realities of life, they live in a dream world. When you tell the average sick person that all their physical troubles are due to a " DIRTY, FILTHY BLOOD STREAM ", how sensitive and insulted they get. They want a careful diagnosis, they want all the modern tests . . . and then the dear ones want a special name given to their physical trouble or troubles. Then they want special treatments for their pet trouble. They still want to smoke, drink alcoholic beverages, tea, coffee, soft and cola drinks, and eat dead, demineralised, devitaminised, bleached, refined foods; also foods empty of calories, BUT, they still want their aches and pains banished.

THERE ARE NO MIRACLE CURES . . . EXCEPT THE MIRACLE CURES THAT NATURE PERFORMS

There is the Great Law of Compensation. You cannot get something for nothing. Health, and I speak of the higher health, must be earned . . . NO ONE CAN CURE YOU . . . NO ONE CAN BANISH YOUR AILMENT. Health is working with this great Law of Compensation . . . Health building requires individual discipline. Your mind and brain must take over the operation of your body. FLESH IS DUMB. You can put anything into your mouth and swallow it.

Only a clear, intelligent and reasoning mind will carefully supervise what is put in the stomach. Remember what you eat today will be walking and talking tomorrow.

The human body is a most powerful instrument and can take years and years of the most cruel punishment. Then comes the day of restitution . . . the human body reaches its capacity for being loaded down with foodless foods that produce a dirty, filthy blood stream. Then disease strikes with all its powerful force and fury. Cataracts blind and blur the vision . . . arthritis cripples and stiffens . . . ears go deaf . . . varicose veins cripple the legs . . . ulcers form in the stomach and intestines, piles, deadly fissures attack the rectum . . . these are just a few of over 4,000 crippling diseases that can make life a living hell on earth.

These tragic things do not just happen . . . it is again the Laws of Compensation working. Disease is not like a thief in the night that creeps up on you and attacks you. YOU—no one else but YOU CREATED THE HORRIBLE Condition that is tormenting your every waking hour. These people who have, through ignorance or through wilfulness brought themselves to this wretched condition physically, will cry out in pain and anguish, " Save me, save me from my suffering and torment ". But I am awfully sorry to inform them there is no one or no treatment that can restore them to health and peace of mind, except the cures Mother Nature provides.

Mother Nature is a hard person to do business with . . . disobey her laws and she will give you punishment that is almost beyond human comprehension. Go to any hospital and see the poor, wretched, suffering humans writhing on their beds of pain. These are the people who never learned the great laws of the care of the human body. Many of them scoffed when well-meaning relatives and friends suggested that they should have a better plan of eating. They were not going to give up their fun . . . so they smoked, drank alcohol, tea, coffee, cola and soft drinks and loaded on refined and dead foods to their hearts content. If you tried to correct their ways, they had all kinds of excuses and answers to cover up their dietetic sins . . . " I am healthy " . . . they would boast . . . " my grandmother lived to be ninety-eight and smoked, drank and ate what she liked. I will be like my old grandmother ". But it did not work out that way . . . now on the hospital bed they were helpless, broken humans ready for the human scrap heap.

Tell me what you eat and I will tell you what you are.

12

YOU MUST DECIDE WHICH ROAD YOU ARE GOING TO TAKE

Your health . . . the length of time you are going to remain on the top of this earth, is strictly up to YOU and YOU alone . . . YOU MUST MAKE THE CHOICE!   You can travel the road that the average person takes and no one will stop you in destroying yourself.   You will have a lot of company.   The average person takes their health for granted.   They want the big thrills of life, or what they think are the big thrills . . . they do not have a correct sense of real values.   " I live it up ", is their cry, " eat what agrees with you ", they say.

But again let me give you a serious warning . . . remember you are going to pay dearly for every dietetic and hygienic sin you commit against your body.   The wages of sin is physical suffering . . . death!

WE MUST NOT CLOG THE PIPES OF THE HUMAN BODY

Our body is really a great plumbing system . . . we are made up of little pipes, medium sized pipes and large pipes like the gastro-intestinal tract, which is thirty feet long.   Throughout the gastro-intestinal pipe from the mouth to the rectum, flow the food and drink we consume.

There is a great muscular system within the gastro-intestinal tract that propels the food down and outward.   To keep this muscular action efficient, the food we eat must contain bulk, moisture and lubrication.   This is supplied by the coarse raw vegetables such as cabbage, carrots, beetroot and celery . . . there are others such as turnips, radishes and squash.   All raw vegetables contribute to strengthen the muscular action along the gastro-intestinal tract.   Raw vegetables and raw fruits are called " Nature's Broom ".   They are absolutely necessary if you are going to enjoy the higher Health.

In my opinion, every disease, no matter what name it is known by scientifically, is basically . . .

CLOGGING OF THE HUMAN PIPE SYSTEM

Any localized symptom is therefore merely an extraordinary local clogging by the accumulated toxic poisons at this particular point.   Any part of the pipe system can become clogged.   The greatest killer of them all, is " Heart Disease ".   The accumulation of foreign toxic matter can clog the arteries of the heart itself.

13

One of the most deadly diseases in the world is hardening of the arteries.

The vicious toxic material that hardens the arteries can completely block them so that your life-giving, oxygenated blood cannot pass through.

Hardening of the arteries does not happen overnight; it takes a long time to bring on this fatal condition. It is said by authoritative sources that some people start to get hardening of the arteries at a very early age.

This was definitely proved during the Korean War where 350 soldiers were closely examined after death. These were young men between the ages of eighteen and twenty-eight. The examination revealed that every one of them had a certain amount of hardening in their arteries. These young men had, since childhood, been fed on highly refined white sugar and refined white sugar products such as cereals, cakes, pies, buns, bread, ice cream, soft drinks, cola drinks, candy and many other products that were heavily saturated with refined white sugar. Many doctors agree that refined white sugar is one of the causes of heart conditions and contributes to the hardening of the arteries. These young men all their life had been fed on commercially hardened fats of all kinds. They were heavy users of salt . . . Salt is a deadly inorganic substance and contains no organic minerals, vitamins, enzymes or nutrients.

They had been fed all the smoked and brine (concentrated salt) cured meats such as bacon, ham, sausage, luncheon meats and all the preserved meats.

In other words they had eaten all the toxic poison producing foods. And as a consequence had started to develop a degenerating disease before they were even thirty.

Just remember that clogging of the human pipe system starts at a very early age. This is the reason why people are biologically older than their chronological age. As I travel over the world I find many people who are twenty to thirty years **older** than their chronological age.

Study the people who are close to you: first look at their foreheads and see how many veins pop out like small snakes . . . look at their hands, see how they have large protruding veins and in many instances their hands and even their faces are filled with dark brown spots. Many are quite deaf, many have poor vision, and many have slow reflexes . . . they move slowly and they think slowly.

These people may be in their forties, fifties or sixties, but they are years and years older than their calendar years, prematurely old and all brought on by obstructions and clogging in the internal pipe system. Their bodies are soaked and saturated with vicious, poisonous toxic material.

Because a person lives to be in their sixties, seventies, eighties or nineties it is no reason that they should suffer from a degenerative disease such as hardening of the arteries. Most people's thinking is controlled by mob psychology. The average person has been trained to think as the years go by, that you are supposed to get older. You are supposed to have deterioration in your body . . . age brings on troubles . . . that is what they have been told and this is exactly what they believe.

You cannot control your chronological years but with the Toxicless Diet Body Purification and Healing System, you can most assuredly control your biological age . . . in fact you can almost hold it to a standstill.

AGELESSNESS

In my opinion, I believe that it is possible to live in a perfect state of agelessness. Let's reason it out together. Every three months you get an entirely new blood stream, so it is not the blood stream that gets old. Every eleven months, every cell in the body has renewed itself . . . so you have practically a new body every eleven months. Every two years you get an entirely new bone structure, so in three years you are really born again . . . the renewal process has taken place. Now, if you keep the body clean and purified by eating a diet that continually keeps purifying the body, how can you get sick? How can you get old? The only thing that can kill you is a disease, time cannot kill you.

I have met in my many years of travels, hundreds of people 100 and more years old; their eyes were perfect, they had no hardening of the arteries, no blindness, no aches and pains. These people lived their early life on farms, they never ate refined and processed foods, but they lived on foods that were close to nature.

If these people had known about the Toxicless Diet Body Purification and Healing System they could control their life indefinitely.

WHY DIE ?

We read in the Bible where people lived to be 900 and more years of age. Of course the sceptics will scoff at these ages and say " They recorded time differently then than we do ". They will tell you it would be impossible to live to be 900. But they have not studied these people's habits. They lived on foods that did not obstruct and clog the pipe system. This was the only thing that kept them alive . . . a clean body, free from clogging, incumbrances and obstructions.

And that is exactly what this Course of Instructions is going to give you. A Way of Life that will help you keep the toxic poisons flushing out of the body. Who knows, you as the reader of this Course of Instructions may live 100 or more years.

Remember that death is brought to the body when it is so saturated and bogged down with toxic poison that it can no longer function. Control the poisons and you control your life.

THE GARDEN OF EDEN

I believe man once lived in a Tropical Paradise. In all my research and study I have come to the definite conclusion that man once lived in a Garden of Eden, and his diet consisted of raw and cooked fruits and vegetables. I believe that the man of Eden ate many green leafed vegetables, I believe he ate nuts and seeds. This is the diet I believe man lived, in freedom of disease and that he lived to be as old as 900 years, or more.

Now I want to clarify this whole statement so I will not be misunderstood. I believe that man lived in this tropical paradise and that at no time did he have to worry about being cold, yes, he lived unclothed and could lie down at night nude and sleep without any discomfort of being cold. This is the true state of man. But then we find this was to change because of the approach of the Ice Ages. All over the world temperatures were altered and varied many times by these Ages. Man was then forced to live in colder climates, his selection and variety of fruits and vegetables was naturally reduced and limited.

Now allow me to repeat for the benefit of emphasis and to make it quite clear in your minds, that while man lived in his tropical paradise, on a diet of naturally grown fruits and vegetables, he was constantly detoxifying and purifying his body. In other words he lived every day on the Toxicless Diet Body Purification and Healing System. He lived for many, many years, free from aches and pains, diseases, premature ageing and senility. But, when he left the Garden of Eden it necessitated his venturing into differing climates, whereby his diet was changed by necessity to the eating of more grain foods like wheat, barley, oats, rye, maize and millet. He also learned to cultivate rice, lentils and

16

beans of all varieties which he dried and stored for long period of time. Having his fruit and vegetable selection greatly reduced, he therefore turned to the killing of animals for meat and the collecting of birds' eggs. In time he found he could domesticate animals like the cow, goat and fowl. Not only did these provide him with ready meat, but he also had fresh eggs supplied and it wasn't long before he mastered the milking of the cow, goat and the sheep.

From this milk he learned to make butter, cheese and other dairy products. So, from a preponderance of an alkaline diet, man was to slowly change his eating habits till his diet was one, heavy in starch and acids. Meat is very heavy in that very toxic acid known as uric acid. Meat is mostly protein, but also carries in it, visible and invisible fats (waxy substance called cholesterol), also the waste that was in circulation through the body at the time of slaughter, not to mention the many viruses and germs of the various animal diseases.

As I travel over the world and study the eating habits of the people, I am bound to make comparisons. Let us take the Eskimo—the Eskimo lives in the frigid Arctic and his diet is almost exclusively animal flesh and the blood of animals and fish. His environment gives him no other recourse for survival than to eat heavily on meat products. These people have a short life span, and they are not particularly attractive people—they age prematurely and in the latter part of their life they suffer from stiff joints, bad livers, bad kidneys and in many instances skin diseases.

NOW, as we move down from the Arctic Circle into the countries like Lapland, Finland and the Northern European countries, we find people using lots of meat, lots of fish, eggs and bread. We get a crystal clear picture of what these foods do to these people. We see premature ageing in these countries, we see the loss of sight, hearing and the general deterioration of the body by the time they have reached sixty. They lose their teeth and many suffer from pyorrhoea. Many have suffered their whole lifetime with some nagging ailment, such as bronchitis, asthma, skin diseases and many other diseases. We go on down into the tropics, and find that people who live in the tropics do not have the know how of eating, that the original people I spoke about had in the Garden of Eden. We find people in the tropics eating lots of pork, fowl, eggs and white rice. In other words, although they live in the tropics they have lost the instinct of living on the Toxicless Diet Body Purification and Healing System, and in the tropics we find lots of disease among these

eprosy, which is one of the most deadly of all

nto what we call the modern twentieth century
, and what do we find, people eat lots of meat; not
ut all kinds of smoked and brine (concentrated salt)
~~cured meat~~ find the civilized people eat many products made from refined white sugar, refined white flour, white rice and processed cheeses. They are using over 2800 chemical additives to colour, preserve and stabilize their foodless foods. The worst crime of all against civilized man's food is the spraying of injurious insecticides, such as arsenic, and many other powerful, deadly chemicals. In his utter despair when he sees his teeth rotting in his head and those of his children, he starts to put deadly fluorides in his drinking water.

And oh, what a sick, broken down creature he is. He has Hospitals, Doctors, Nurses, Bacteriologists, Phamaceutical Researchers and Chemists trying to do something to help him in his misery. In the United States, which is a representative country of these so-called civilized countries, 47 times in every second a prescription is filled by a white coated chemist at one of the 56,000 Chemist-Drug Shops in the United States. The staggering cost of these pink, violet, yellow, white and green tablets, capsules, lozenges and ampules, amounts to over $14 billion a year.

MAN IS SICK, and has been for a long time, and is getting sicker. It has almost reached a point of total helplessness.

Not only are the adults sick in body, but they are sick in mind. 30% of the hospital beds in our civilized countries are used up by people suffering from some mental condition. Nearly one out of ten children is born either a cripple or retarded—the insane asylums of the civilized world are packed to overflowing.

This is a long way that man has come from the Garden of Eden where he lived on the clean purifying foods, enjoying perfect health, and many long years of happy life.

"WE CANNOT GO BACK TO THE GARDEN OF EDEN"

I want you to know I have no illusions that there is any place left in the world that could be called a Garden of Eden. Man, if he wants to be well and live long, must create his own Garden of Eden wherever he is.

That is exactly what the Toxicless Diet Body Purification and Healing System is going to do, it's going to help you establish wherever you are—your own Garden of Eden! We cannot expect to have the health and the vitality and the long life that our brothers and

"Most of the mentally retarded babies born in America are due to poor eating habits where the mother lacked the basic nutrients (vitamins and minerals) needed to produce a healthy baby!"

—Dr. Roger Williams, Noted Scientist & Nutritionist

sisters enjoyed in their Garden of Eden. But we can, by careful control of our diet, purify our bodies by flushing out of our bodies the vicious toxic poisons that are causing us suffering.

Naturally there will be a lot of compromises made. We have had many generations of evolution in eating an unbalanced diet, so now we begin our journey back to the Garden of Eden slowly and cautiously.

FIRST STEP IN THE TOXICLESS DIET BODY PURIFICATION AND HEALING SYSTEM

The beginning of this programme must start with your avoiding the foods and drinks that clog, obstruct, and throw waste into the human pipe system, into the organs of the body and the cells. Study the following list of so-called foods, drinks, and other materials and never again, ever let them pass through your body.

They work slowly, but very effectively and are deadly. The first thirty-five—forty years of life most people can wilfully or ignorantly attempt to break the laws of human bio-chemistry. Some people have stronger constitutions than others, so people will often make this statement to me—" My Grandfather is eighty-eight and smokes, drinks alcohol, and eats any food he wants to, and still he is living". I have to listen to this occasionally because there are the lucky few who inherit a body that has wide arteries and wide veins, and are born with a capacity to burn poisons three times faster than the average person. But just remember this, when a person eighty-eight was born, there were 86,000 others, and he is the lone survivor. One out of 86,000—so that's not a very good percentage.

Now, on the other hand, if that man had known about the Toxicless Diet Body Purification and Healing System that had kept toxic materials down to a minimum, who knows, he might have lived to be 150. I have met many men and women from 125—135 years of age and I was able to check out their ages authentically by records, wills and other legal documents.

So the first thing to do is to discard forever the following so-called foods and materials which humans put into their bodies. . .

FOODS TO AVOID

* Refined sugar or refined sugar products such as jams, jellies, preserves, marmalade, ice cream, sherberts, Jello, cake, candy, cookies, chewing gum, soft drinks, pies, pastries, tapioca puddings, sugared fruit juices, fruits canned in sugar syrup.

AVOID THESE PROCESSED, REFINED, HARMFUL FOODS

Once you realize the irreparable harm caused to your body by refined, chemicalized, deficient foods, it is not difficult to eat correctly. Simply eliminate these "killer" foods from your diet...and follow an eating plan which provides the basic, essential nourishment your body needs.

- Refined sugar or refined sugar products such as jams, jellies, preserves, marmalades, yogurts, ice cream, sherberts, Jello, cake, candy, cookies, chewing gum, soft drinks, pies, pastries, tapioca puddings, sugared fruit juices & fruits canned in sugar syrup.

- Salted foods, such as corn chips, salted crackers, salted nuts

- Catsup & mustard w/salt-sugar, Worchestershire sauce, pickles, olives

- White rice & pearled barley   • Fried & greasy foods

- Commercial, highly processed dry cereals such as corn flakes, etc.

- Saturated fats & hydrogenated oils...(heart enemies that clog bloodstream)

- Food which contains palm & cottonseed oil. Products labeled vegetable oil...find out what kind, before you use it.

- Oleo & margarines...(saturated fats & hydrogenated oils)

- Peanut butter that contains hydrogenated, hardened oils

- Coffee, decaffeinated coffee, China black tea & all alcoholic beverages

- Fresh pork & pork products   • Fried, fatty & greasy meats

- Smoked meats, such as ham, bacon & sausage, smoked fish

- Luncheon meats, such as hot dogs, salami, bologna, corned beef, pastrami & any packaged meats containing dangerous sodium nitrate or nitrite

- Dried fruits containing sulphur dioxide - a preservative

- Do not eat chickens that have been injected with stilbestrol, or fed with chicken feed that contains any drug

- Canned soups - read labels for sugar, starch, white, wheat flour & preservatives

- Food that contains benzoate of soda, salt, sugar, cream of tartar...& any additives, drugs or preservatives

- White flour products such as white bread, wheat-white bread, enriched flours, rye bread that has wheat-white flour in it, dumplings, biscuits, buns, gravy, noodles, pancakes, waffles, soda crackers, macaroni, spaghetti, pizza, ravioli, pies, pastries, cakes, cookies , prepared and commercial puddings, and ready-mix bakery products. (Health Stores have a huge variety of 100% whole grain products.)

- Day-old, cooked vegetables & potatoes, & pre-mixed old salads

SECOND STEP IN THE TOXICLESS DIET BODY PURIFICATION AND HEALING SYSTEM

First thing you do before you go on this diet is to sit down and carefully analyse yourself. You know how you feel, no one in the world could diagnose in detail your problems, therefore you must do a little self diagnosing. You have read the list of clogging and toxic forming foods and you know within your own heart how many dietetic indiscretions you have made, and over how many years.

So you balance your ailments against your diet—you may have had bronchitis or asthma for many, many years—all this is to be taken into consideration before you can live completely on the Toxicless Diet Body Purification and Healing System. You've got to consider if you have had any operations, you've got to consider how many drugs you have used, because you not only have to get the food poison out of your system, but if you have used drugs of any kind, they too are buried deeply into the tissues and must be flushed out!

The next consideration is how far your vitality has been lowered, and just how much vital force still remains in your body. The more physical troubles you have had over your life, the more drugs you have taken, so all this will have to be taken into consideration. How much meat do you eat, how many eggs do you eat, how much dairy products do you eat . . . these will all have to be carefully considered. After these have been carefully considered you are ready to establish for yourself the third step in the programme.

THIRD STEP IN THE TOXICLESS DIET BODY PURIFICATION AND HEALING SYSTEM—YOUR INDIVIDUAL TRANSITION DIET

I want you to remember first, and keep it in mind at all times, that the ideal diet of man is raw and cooked fruit, raw and baked vegetables, nuts and seeds, with a preponderance of raw and cooked green leafed vegetables (chard, spinach, beetroot tops, turnip greens, mustard greens, collards, kale, etc.). I do not expect you, unless you are very ambitious about a thorough internal cleansing, to try to reach the ideal state of purification. There are various degrees of health that can be obtained by controlling the diet. I feel that if a person can in time balance the diet to 50% raw fruits and vegetables and properly cooked fruits and vegetables, and with a minimum amount of protein, fats, natural sugars and natural starches, they can live in a very high state of health and have many long, vigorous years.

The Transition Diet starts first with a total water fast of twenty-four hours, nothing is passed through the body in this twenty-four hours except water. Fasting IS the greatest of all detoxifiers because when we stop eating all the vital force that was used to masticate, digest and assimilate the food and eliminate the waste is used to purify the body. All this powerful energy is now released to flush the accumulated obstructions and toxic poisons from the body. After the fast of twenty-four hours you make it an iron firm rule always to begin every meal with something raw. This will re-educate the two hundred and sixty taste buds of your mouth to the delicate natural flavour of raw foods. Of course this cannot be obtained if a person smokes either a cigarette, cigar or pipe, because nicotine completely paralyses the taste buds, so the Transition Diet is wasted completely on a smoker. The same goes for alcohol, tea, coffee, soft drinks and cola drinks. So please eliminate smoking and also these beverages from your diet. Salt must also be entirely eliminated on this cleansing diet and from this day on—use no salt!

STEP FOUR OF THE TOXICLESS DIET BODY PURIFICATION AND HEALING SYSTEM

The healing crisis is one of the great mysteries of the Toxicless Diet Body Purification and Healing System. Most humans have been so inculcated with the idea that when you have something wrong with you and you want to improve your health, you go and get a physical examination—you are diagnosed—and then a name may be given to your ailment. The person then is put under treatment and he feels that under this treatment he is going to feel better and stronger, and if he is sick that he is going to get well. Now, don't expect to feel this way in the Toxicless Diet Body Purification and Healing System. As you start on this System of Purification you are going to stir up old toxic poisons, and you do have plenty of them. Everyone else also has them, because most everyone carries from five—ten pounds of deeply buried toxic poisons in their bodies at all times. That is the reason it is so ridiculous when I hear people say " I am healthy ". When they make that statement to me I say " Let me put you on a ' fast ' followed by the Toxicless Diet Body Purification and Healing System and I'll show you how much of these deeply buried poisons you have stored in your body ".

That is what sickness is in the final analysis—the body becomes so corroded and loaded with vicious toxic poisons that it throws up its own healing crisis, in the form of a cold, flu, pneumonia, boils, abscesses and hundreds of other manifestations of the body ridding itself of poisons. Disease is no mystery to me, it does not come like a thief in the night, it is something that is slowly built up to by toxic poisons in every organ of the body.

So be ready for a series of healing crises if you expect to attain vitality supreme. This is a compensation action—this is the Vital Force asserting itself. You cannot get away from paying your price to Mother Nature, there is no way to circumvent the crimes you have committed against your body.

I am not going to tell you that when you go on the Transition Diet along with your twenty-four-hour weekly fast, and by eating more fruits and vegetables in the diet and eliminating some of the heavier foods, that you are going to feel good right away. You will not feel your best until you have eliminated a large amount of the toxic poisons from your body.

I do not give special diets for special ailments. I don't believe in curative diets. I believe that you must slowly, through fasting and eating more raw fruits and vegetables, flush out the heavy accumulation of toxic poisons.

STEP FIVE OF THE TOXICLESS DIET BODY PURIFICATION AND HEALING SYSTEM

Our bodies are fine instruments and the cleaner they become through the Toxicless Diet Body Purification and Healing System they will absorb first, more oxygen which is the source of all life. A toxic filled body can only take so much oxygen because it is encumbered with so many obstructions. As you purify your body you will feast on the invisible foods of the universe, your body will absorb more oxygen, more electricity, more ozone, more of the sun's strength-giving rays. Think of it—living on the invisible foods of nature. Babies do this—they eat only a small amount of food and mother's milk is only $3\frac{1}{2}\%$ protein. But, did you ever watch a healthy active baby kick and wiggle and coo for hours at a time? Where is the energy coming from . . . not from the Mother's milk with only $3\frac{1}{2}\%$ protein. That baby's body is so clean that it has gathered from the universe the powerful nutrition that is invisible. Look at the baby's skin, how delicate; look at his wide, bright eyes and at his sunny smile, and at his powerful lungs when he cries.

23

Now look at a person of seventy-five and look at their wrinkled, crepey, miserable looking flesh, their eyes may be covered with cataracts, they are almost human caricatures. Don't tell me it is because the man is seventy-five and the baby is five months. The difference is that the old man has been soaking up toxic poisons for most of the years of his life and this is toxemia —this is the result of clogging, this is the result of a life-long intake of toxic forming foods.

MOVE WITH CAUTION—VITALITY FROM
THE UNIVERSE

A man at seventy-five could really have only lived half of his lifetime, and I support this statement by the fact that every other animal lives from five—seven times his rate of maturity. A number of years ago I had a pet dog which was in pup. Determined to have the healthiest litter possible, I fed my old dog a balanced nutritional diet. There was only one pup born and I called him " Vitamin ". When born he was an exceptionally healthy and beautiful pup and I made sure I kept him that way throughout his 154 years of life, by feeding him only with the most nutritional diets available. As a consequence my " Vitamin " won many first prizes, at dog shows all over the world. Yes, "Vitamin" did live to be 154 years of age, in ratio to human years. His actual years lived were twenty-two. You see, in relation to the human span, a dog's year lived is equivalent to seven years lived by a human. Even at this age he was still quite a healthy dog. Sorrowfully though for me, he died in his twenty-second year, when three dogs ganged up on him and killed him.

If I can only burn into your consciousness that toxic poisons and wastes are the encumbrances that deteriorate human flesh, but that doesn't mean an old skin.

Naturally an adult that lives an active life in the sun and the fresh air is going to have a more matured skin than a five months' old baby.

I have seen men and women in their eighties and nineties who did not have a wrinkle in their face, nor a line nor any drying tissue. The last time I saw the famous Doctor John Harvey Kellogg, one of the greatest American doctors that ever lived, he was in his ninety-third year and he was giving a lecture on health. The thing that impressed me so much about Dr. Kellogg was that he had the skin of a young baby, he had no wrinkles, no lines, no dehydrating, crepey skin, he had a round, smooth face with the glow of health shining through.

PEOPLE I HAVE KNOWN WHO REFUSE TO GROW OLD

In my professional work as a Dietetic Advisor to the Film Stars of Hollywood, I have many women who absolutely defy time because they have learned the Toxicless Diet Body Purification and Healing System. You could never determine their age because at fifty they look thirty and the woman of sixty looks and acts like forty.

The outward signs of this age-defying youthfulness are a straight-backed posture, supple breast contours, taut smooth skin on face and neck, firm muscles and that particular vigour and grace, typical of a healthy female. At fifty such women still look attractive in tennis shorts or sleeveless dresses.

To the emotionally mature woman, this physical attractiveness is rarely an end in itself, rather, it's a subtle, psychological means by which she relates to the world around her. While this quality may not be directly erotic, its charm is usually derived from a woman's sexual self-confidence. Now, thanks to the Toxicless Diet Body Purification and Healing System, it is possible for any woman to retain her sexual appeal, as well as her sexual vitality throughout later life. By retaining these functions she also safeguards a less direct and more allusive aspect of her total feminity.

The way of getting old-looking can be a thing of the past for any woman who will take the time and the discipline to purify her body, and I do believe that through body purification women can remain youthful and feminine forever!

And that goes for men too. We know that women do have a better sense of taking care of themselves, so that they may look younger and wear their clothes with grace and charm, and that most men destroy themselves with tobacco, alcohol and a heavy acid meat diet. It is a well-known fact that women live anywhere from five—ten years longer than the average man. She just does not have the capacity or the inclination to eat heavy, greasy meat meals. To the average man a big steak and a large pile of fried potatoes is good eating, and that's the reason that men are dying off from forty to fifty in alarming numbers. The civilized world is full of widows simply because most men scoff or ridicule the idea of following a programme of good nutrition.

I have men in the T.V. and movie picture profession who through my consultation and advice have been able to retain a boyish figure, a youthful voice, even though they are in their sixties. They feel and act twenty years younger, or more, than their actual age. The same with a non-professional man. I have men students who are in their sixties and seventies who look in their thirties and forties.

One of the most outstanding men in the world who has carefully followed the natural health life is Robert Cummings, the distinguished American actor and T.V. star, author and lecturer—a man who has reached his sixties and still retains the youthful look of a man in his early thirties.

Most men are dietetic sinners; left to their own resources they will try to live on a ham, egg, toast, steak and fried potato diet. This is the reason our obituary columns are filled with the death notices of men in their forties, fifties and sixties.

Not only do these men die young, but through either ignorance or wilfulness, they will not follow the principles of nutrition, thus they suffer from many ailments. Most men living on this one-sided toxic diet, lose their Adam Power very early in life. I have men in their thirties and forties complaining of being totally impotent—many of these men have a diseased prostate gland that finally has to be surgically removed. The average man about forty in our civilized environment today is a candidate for a heart attack, suffering from some chronic disease and an early death. He is also a candidate for prostate surgery.

The Doctors' offices of the civilized world are filled with women who suffer at their menstrual period, and in the United States seven out of ten women reaching sixty have had some type of surgery on the female organs.

TOXIC POISONS CAUSE IMPOTENT MEN AND FRIGID WOMEN

No wonder in the civilized countries our divorce rate is staggering. Impotent men, frigid women, cannot hold up their end of the marital relationship. Most divorces in our civilized countries are caused by physical incompatability, so we can see that when toxic poisons get into the reproductive glands of both male and female, serious ailments take place. When you suffer with toxic poisons in those organs—the sexual desires diminish more and more as the toxins build up.

There is no reason why, biologically, man and woman cannot retain their sexual energies up to ninety and longer. The only thing that can happen to the reproductive organs of both man and woman is a diseased condition which is brought on by the person's ignorance in the science of total living.

Remember, we are punished by our bad habits of living, and we are rewarded by our good habits of living.

INTERNAL COSMETICS WHEN YOU GO ON THE TOXICLESS DIET BODY PURIFICATION AND HEALING SYSTEM

Progressively eliminate the greater portions of the heavy foods from your diet and eat more fruits and vegetables and you will notice the skin and muscle tone changing. There is a complete rejuvenation. Fruits and vegetables are the Internal Cosmetics which reveal their wonderful working power in giving you a healthy glowing skin.

So you see, in going on the Toxicless Diet Body Purification and Healing System there are so many things that you are rewarded with—first you eliminate your obstructions, toxic poisons, and your aches and pains and miseries. Your energy is lifted to a high degree, you no longer suffer from fatigue and excessive tiredness—the changes are miraculous.

A NEW YOU IS CREATED EVERY DAY

When you faithfully follow the Toxicless Diet Body Purification and Healing System the changes you see in the mirror sometimes of yourself will startle you. When you first go on it and start the elimination process, sometimes you will look wretched. This usually happens during the crisis period, when the greatest amount of poisons are loosened from the pipes and vital organs and are being flushed out of the body. When you have gone through the crisis several times then you can see the New You revealing itself. The eyes become brighter, the skin muscle tone becomes very healthy, the joints of the body are more supple and there is a state of well being that throbs throughout your entire body that makes you glad you are alive.

Each day when you live on the Toxicless Diet Body Purification and Healing System you make changes and adjustments in your body, but they are always good adjustments and you are creating a stronger body, a well body, a vigorous body and a healthy body. To me it's worth all the effort, all the hard work that must go into living by this natural way of life, which man has strayed from due to the commercial, over-civilized world we live in.

As I have stated, to what degree of physical perfection you wish to attain is solely a personal matter with you.

You must remember that fifty—sixty per cent of the diet should be made up of raw fruits and vegetables and properly cooked fruits and vegetables. Your protein, plus your natural sugars, plus your natural oils, plus your natural starches and carbohydrates should compose the balance.

I must remind you again that I have no special diets for special ailments, I believe there is only one cause for all ailments, and that is internal clogging. When we can break and flush out of the body these vicious obstructions, then you are on the Royal Road to Health.

IT TAKES FROM TWO TO THREE YEARS TO REACH THE HIGH POINT IN INTERNAL PERFECTION

Keep in mind CONSTANTLY it took quite a long time to get in the condition you are in now, through wrong habits and wrong eating, and now you must be patient with nature, you cannot throw caution to the wind. If you have been used to eating meat several times a day, and eggs every day and cheese every day, you have to slowly eliminate the excessive use of these foods.

As you fast one day a week, and as you add more fruits and vegetables to your diet, you will soon estimate how much of the stimulating foods that you can eat every day, and gradually you reach a status quo. This is the point where no longer toxic poisons are retained in the body, this is the time you reach a peak of internal fitness, a point of perfection, and this is the condition everyone should seek—they should be able to eat a balanced diet and still maintain a Clean, Painless, Tireless, Ageless Body.

CAUTION—MOVE SLOWLY

Keep in mind always " the wheels of the Gods move slowly but surely ". You can't push nature, you can't be impatient and expect to reach a perfect state of internal fitness in a few months.

STEP SIX IN THE TOXICLESS DIET BODY PURIFICATION AND HEALING SYSTEM

My experiences of over seventy years, covering the most extreme severe cases of all kinds of physical problems, has proven that a carefully selected and progressively changed transition diet is the best way for every person to obtain their goal. As long as foodless foods (refined foods of civilization) are partially used you must not overdo on too much fresh fruit and fresh vegetables. Also every person must learn, if they want to attain biochemical perfection, that they should not eat a regular morning breakfast. You will continually hear people say " breakfast is the most important meal of the day ",—this is not true— scientifically it takes a tremendous amount of nervous energy to masticate, digest, assimilate and eliminate a regular breakfast. Now, let us say a person gets up in the morning with the idea that if they eat a hearty breakfast it's going to give them strength. Most average people believe this, being told by the producers of cereals, breads, eggs, tea, coffee, cocoa, milk—this is propaganda by these big powerful interests. It is to their interest to brainwash people into believing they should have this big breakfast and that it is just going to fill them full of energy.

Let's look at it from a cold, scientific viewpoint. If you eat a breakfast of cold or hot cereal, two eggs, bacon, three slices of buttered toast and some beverage like tea or coffee, it is not immediately converted into strength and energy. You must realize this, that it takes a great deal of time and energy for the stomach and digestive system to mix this (not needed, heavy breakfast) food, with the various digestive juices for the slow process of mastication, digestion and assimilation. Then the separation process takes place, the proteins in the stomach are to be digested by their special digestive juices, the starches, sugars and fats are pushed out into the small intestine for the digestion of these special nutrients.

Foods of all categories have special juices to digest them. All foods need a large amount of enzymes to break them down so that they can be sent into the blood stream. This all takes many hours—some people have very slow digestions. After all this hard digestive work has been done in the digestive tract, breaking this food down into a fine liquid, it has to pass through the intestines, past little organs known as " villi ". They are along the digestive tract and as the liquified food substance passes by them, they have little suckers that draw the nourishment into the blood.

AGAIN let me emphasize that this takes hours—so if anyone tells you you get immediate strength from eating breakfast you know they are totally ignorant of the facts of digestion.

You may say to me, "Yes, that's very well but I'm hungry in the morning, I get up hungry" and I will have to answer you and say "You are all wrong—the stomach has been conditioned to load up with food in the morning, and so, what you mistake for hunger is simply a reflex action built up by a long habit of eating break-fast ". Once you discard breakfast and live on the " no breakfast " plan, you could never again put a heavy amount of food into your stomach again in the morning.

The morning is the time to drink fresh fruit juices, or better still eat the whole fresh fruit. This is the ideal nourishment for early morning, because fruit requires the most infinitesimal amount of digestion and the natural sugars of fresh fruit can give you more blood sugar energy than eggs, meat, toast, buns, and sausage. Your body operates on blood sugar—a healthy person manufactures about a fourth of a cup daily and this blood sugar is where the muscles draw their energy from. Fruit is light and does not require the tremendous amount of nervous energy to digest that cereals, meat, eggs and other heavy foods require.

I have seen people go on the " no breakfast " plan alone, along with a good diet, with plenty of raw fruits and vegetables, and they have banished many physical problems.

MIRACLES WITHIN YOUR POWER

Now you can get a bird's eye view of the Toxicless Diet Body Purification and Healing System—the " no breakfast " plan, complete water fast one day weekly and the progressive adding of more raw fruits, more raw vegetables and more properly cooked fruits and vegetables. When you reach this point, then you will see the New You appear! You will feel different, you will have more energy, endurance, you will sleep easier and you will wake up in the morning well rested. The nagging aches and pains that have troubled you will fade away. Your eyes will become clear, your skin will have a more youthful tone to it . . . these are the rewards—these are the high rewards you receive by putting yourself totally in the hands of Mother Nature and living by her great laws.

TRANSITION DIET FULLY EXPLAINED

I want you to understand thoroughly that the Toxicless Diet Body Purification and Healing System is not made up of special diets for specific ailments. There are no special diets given. It is based on a System of Eating, that first eliminates the deep buried toxic poison, obstructions and encumbrances that have been in the body for years. If drugs have been taken, the concentrations of these drugs are still buried deep in the spongy organs of the body and they must be removed before causing trouble.

During the time I was suffering with T.B. I was given enormous amounts of powerful drugs. It took five years for me to eliminate those drugs from my tissues. I went through a number of crises before I was at last free from vicious drug poison.

The Toxicless Diet Body Purification and Healing System goes directly to the cause of your physical problem. The System has no interest in the effects of a basic cause. Most people want the symptom of their problem treated or a special diet given.

I believe that all physical problems are caused by an excess of toxic poison in the pipes and organs of the body, therefore I am interested in so eating and fasting that these long buried poisons will be flushed out of the body.

I do not believe that physical problems are caused by over-work, tensions, strains, stresses or emotional upsets. A strong, clean, toxic-free body can meet any of these troubles. Some people will say that all their problems are due to nerves. This is not so. When the nerves are free of toxic poisons they can meet any crises that a human is forced to face.

People with deep-seated physical problems want to blame everything on someone or some imaginary cause. In going on this programme you have to admit that you and you alone are responsible for your physical condition and that you and you alone must battle the situation!

CURE YOURSELF? THAT IS EXACTLY WHAT YOU HAVE TO DO

Some people may have brought on their troubles because they were ignorant of the great Nutritional Laws of Life. Some know that following the Programme of Natural Nutrition is the most important factor in regaining and maintaining health, but they do not have the inner strength to battle their false desires for foodless foods. For they are wilful and persist in building up the toxic poisons in their body through their wrong diet.

Each individual must face the issue that only through their own daily constructive, healthful actions can they HEAL THEM-SELVES!

This is a cold, hard world. There is a price tag on everything in life.

If you want the Higher Health, if you want to prolong your life you must pay the price with hard work, which means following a strict health diet and being consistent with your twenty-four-hour weekly fast.

The energy and vitality of a young child can be yours, at any age. That's what you can do for yourself when you follow this special way of life. This System gives you the vitality of youthful-ness, because that is just exactly what youthfulness is—Internal Purity! It is not a matter of age, it is perfect internal condition.

It is true that in calendar years I am over eighty years young. But this is not my true age. I do not live by calendar years.

I live in biological years. That is what counts. How clean are your arteries and veins? How are your blood pressures? I have blood pressures of 120 over 80. This is the blood pressure of a boy of twenty. I have a steady, strong pulse of sixty. I have the eyes of an eagle and keen ears that can pick up the lightest sounds.

I am not interested in my birthdays. I am concentrating my attention on Internal Purity. And when you seriously follow the Toxicless Diet Body Purification and Healing System you will experience what I am experiencing. You must work at it every day. It is not a fad, it is something that must become a part of you and your daily living. I want to live. I want to feel strong and vigorous every day. I do not want to be plagued with aches and pains.

So, up to this point I eat from fifty to sixty per cent of my food raw—fruits and vegetables and properly cooked fruits and vegetables. I have been able to discard a large amount of the stimulating foods. In other words I am working daily on my Internal Purity.

One step is the beginning of a ten thousand mile journey. As soon as you make the start . . . **YOU** too can start to enjoy the Higher Health!

NOW GO TO WORK ON FLUSHING THE TOXIC POISONS OUT OF YOUR BODY

1. Eliminate forever the toxic foods of civilization (see page 19).

2. Take a complete twenty-four-hour water fast every seven days. My book " The Miracle of Fasting " will give you all the vital information you need to know on this tremendous subject. The back cover will tell you where you can purchase this book.

3. Eliminate breakfast. (If it is too difficult for you to, just do on fruit juice and fresh fruit then you can add raw wheat germ and honey to your fruit.) Some people are so habit-bound to a big breakfast that it takes a little time to eliminate this unimportant meal. If you still feel you need more in your stomach in the morning try a dish of whole-grain cereal, or an egg and a few slices of whole-meal toast. But remember this is the most useless and energy robbing meal of the day.

Have your Apple Cider Vinegar and Honey cocktail* early in the morning. It consists of one tablespoon of natural apple cider vinegar and one tablespoon of natural honey mixed in a glass of water.

*Read the Bragg *Vinegar* book for more information.

When you give up that breakfast you will have ten times the energy you had before. In my own personal life I do my most creative work in the morning. And when I am ready for my physical activity such as hiking, swimming, tennis or sports, I am full of strength to enjoy my activity. It takes a tremendous amount of energy to digest a regular breakfast. You cannot put your energy in two places at once, food and activity. People often wonder why I accomplish so much between 6 a.m. and noon. It is because I have not dissipated my Vital Force on the big breakfast. My cocktail, fruit juice and fresh fruit is all I need and I have inexhaustible energy.

YOU MUST EARN YOUR FOOD

4. By noon you are now ready for the first meal of the day. You have earned it. You have used both mental and physical effort. Always start this first important main meal with a large combination salad, consisting of the broom coarse vegetables—all raw—either chopped or grated, cabbage, carrots, beetroot and celery—they are the base of your health salad. To this combination you can add any raw vegetables you desire. Cucumbers (green skin too), lettuce, radishes, parsley, avocado, tomatoes, green onions or any fresh raw vegetable.

You can make a salad dressing of natural cider vinegar, health salad oil (soya, peanut, safflower, sunflower, sesame or olive oil) and honey. You always eat your fill of raw salad first. Never let hot food touch your mouth until you have had your fill of the raw salad. The salad is the internal purifier. The salad is the fighter of toxic poisons. Toxic poisons just have to move out of the body when the nutrients of the raw salads get to work.

But if you have not been used to eating a large raw vegetable salad, GO SLOWLY. You may say to me, " Raw salad fills me with gas" or "Raw salads do not agree with me". And I must answer " The salads agree with you, but **you** do not agree with the salads ". When a raw salad does not agree with you, it shows you have a mucus condition in the bowel. They are sick bowels. So, there is only one thing to do and that is to move slowly. It took a long time for the bowel to be in this awful condition and it will take time and conditioning to get the bowel ready to accept the raw salads. That is the reason this System is not giving a person a cut and dried diet. Everyone is different. Each person must move at the speed that fits their condition. People with bad

Having heard the word, keep it, and bring forth fruit with patience.
—Luke 8:15

dentures must cut or grate the salad very fine. But remember, the daily salad is very important. It is the master internal cleanser.

5. The next question is what to eat with this salad. The best thing would be a fresh cooked vegetable like a baked potato, string beans, steamed cabbage, peas, corn on the cob, carrots, beetroot, steamed greens or any fresh cooked vegetable you desire.

6. Now what about the protein? If you feel you need meat, eat it. Just remember, on this diet you do not eat meat but three times a week. You can have fresh fish several times a week and then you can have the vegetable proteins such as nuts and seeds.

Now due to bad teeth the nuts would be better ground or taken in the form of nut butters . . . the same with seeds like sunflower or sesame seeds. It may be best to eat them ground.

Many times I have my big raw salad for lunch and I finish off with dried fruits such as dates, raisins, figs and nuts.

7. Don't worry about getting protein. Traces of protein are found in all foods. Just think, a mother's milk is only $3\frac{1}{2}\%$ protein and a new human body is built with this small amount of protein. I never worry about getting my daily quota of protein. The body is a great chemical instrument and can very easily convert any other food to protein. I do not believe in the heavy protein diet. For over forty years I have heard nutritionists declare the great value of a high protein diet. But in my consultation work, I have found many who went on a high protein diet get into serious troubles (high blood pressures, heart trouble, gout, kidney, prostate and liver disorders).

The racehorse does not eat concentrated protein. He gets his great speed, strength and endurance from the vegetable kingdom. Nuts, seeds, raw wheat germ, brewers yeast, natural brown rice, and many dried beans are rich, healthy sources of non-cholesterol, non-uric acid protein.

You must always keep in mind that meat is a second-hand food. The animal ate the green growing things that produced the meat. And when that animal was killed, it retained all the poisons that it had within its body. I have told you that meat has uric acid and it contains heavy concentrations of visible and invisible saturated fats. Remember these are the waxy fats (cholesterol) that clog and plug up the human pipe system and the vital organs.

I know people all over the world eat meat. But in America, Australia, New Zealand and the United Kingdom, they consume large amounts of meats in the daily diet . . . and we also know that one out of every two deaths are caused in these countries by heart attacks. And heart specialists agree that the waxy saturated fats of meat are the main villain by causing clogged arteries and clogged veins.

I never try to make a health student a vegetarian. I believe, by properly combining the natural foods, that people can eat meat three times a week and live a long healthy life. But I believe that the one-sided meat eater does get himself into serious trouble.

I have told you what the ideal diet of man was when he was in the warm tropical Garden of Eden. Now man lives everywhere and he must adapt himself to the climate he is in. I do not believe it is possible for a person who is living in a cold climate to eat as if he lived in the tropics. Unless the fruits and vegetables are available, and he has conditioned his blood stream to the climate, he must eat plenty of nuts and seeds to build a blood stream that will keep him warm.

Remember your diet must fit in with your climate. That does not mean because you live in a cold climate you eat more meat. It means you eat meat three times a week and you eat fresh fish and then you use nuts, seeds, brown rice, raw wheat germ and the dried beans for protein the other days.

But you always keep the basic principle of the System in mind at all times, that you keep adding more raw fruits and vegetables to the diet. Remember the raw fruits and vegetables are the purifiers and the detoxicator.

That is why one-sided meat and starch eaters get into serious troubles. They are eating too much toxic forming foods.

OVER-EATING—A SLOW KILLER

Some people eat as though they were going to do the hardest kind of physical labour. A sedentary person by habit and conditioning will get up in the morning and eat a heavy breakfast of cooked or dried cereal, ham and eggs, buttered toast and a stimulating beverage like tea or coffee or sometimes milk, which is mucus forming. No animal except man ever drinks milk after they are weaned. I do not approve of milk drinking for adults— neither raw nor pasteurized.

They then go to work in an office, store, etc., and sit or stand around. They will usually have a mid-morning snack and at noon they will eat a heavy meal: bread and meat and dessert and again a beverage like tea or coffee. In the mid-afternoon, more snacks and tea or coffee. Then home for the biggest meal of the day; consisting of meat, potatoes, bread, dessert and a beverage, and to top off the day while watching

T.V., will snack again. This kind of daily habit is making tens of thousands of sick people, exhausted people . . . sending them to hospitals and to an early grave.

The average person living the ordinary inactive life cannot possibly burn this tremendous amount of food. So what happens to people who eat this way? You know as well as I do they are sick or half-sick most of their entire lifetimes.

They fill the Chemist-Drug Shops, the mental institutions, the old people's homes and arrive early at the graveyard.

Over-eating is a vicious and dangerous habit, and most people over-eat. They have been told they must have regular meals at regular hours, and they believe this nonsense. They hardly have one meal down before they are putting down another. They think that by this constant stuffing, that they are " keeping up their strength "—they are doing the opposite—they are weakening their Vital Power. Why? By over-eating they are burdening their whole system—also this continual eating never gives the machinery time to repair or rest. Reason I stress a twenty-four-hour weekly fast as a must! This is so vital to unclogging and cleansing your system.

I see these over-stuffed people every day of my life. Most of them suffer from chronic fatigue. They get up tired and go to bed tired. They push all kinds of stimulants into themselves to try and keep going. In civilization today people take pep pills to keep going during the day and sleeping pills to try and get to sleep at night. What a pitiful plight the average person gets himself into.

RIDICULE FOR THOSE WHO WANT BETTER HEALTH

These same half-dead creatures are always ready to say cruel things about those who want to take better care of themselves by Constructive Conscious Control of their bodies.

People like me are called " fanatics ", " food cranks ", " health nuts". The big producers of civilized refined and dead-foods are largely responsible for these curt remarks about people who become vitally interested in good nutrition and natural hygienic living. If living by the wholesome Plan of Nature and God Almighty is being a fanatic . . . then I will lay claim to being the biggest fanatic in this whole wide world. I am proud I live close to God and Nature's Plan of Living. I am jealous of my health, and I intend to protect it until I draw my last breath.

This is the reason why, when you decide to go on the Toxicless Diet Body Purification and Healing System don't tell your

---

The unexamined life is not worth living. It is a time to re-evaluate your past as a guide to your future.

—Socrates

relatives, in-laws or out-laws. It is strictly ⸝
Tell only the ones whom it is absolutely nece
average persons who stuff three big meals
stomachs, think illness, or premature old-age and ᴜᴄᴄ
something no one can control.

These people I call, " the unthinking living dead ". They are
so full of internal corruption . . . they are so toxic, so filled with
internal clogging that there is nothing you can say to them. They
will all follow the same pattern. They will have a flush of youth
in their early years and then they will start to decline.

I never argue with these " living dead ". I never allow myself
to get down to their level mentally. I know what the Toxicless
Diet Body Purification and Healing System has done for me. I
know what it has done for my children, my grandchildren and my
great-grandchildren. Why should I waste my precious energy
trying to convince some toxic-loaded, wilful, ignorant person (who
could care less) the value of good nutrition?

MORE ABOUT THE TRANSITION DIET

8. Now we come to the evening meal. There should always
be at least six hours between each meal. The digestive system
must have time to do its important work efficiently. Again the
evening meal must start with some kind of raw fruit or vegetable
salad. Let us say, for instance, at the noon meal you had a large
raw vegetable salad, so now you would like a different raw salad
. . . maybe you would enjoy just a large cole slaw (grated or
chopped cabbage) salad, or a cabbage and carrot salad or a raw
grated beetroot and cabbage salad. There are so many varieties
of salads a person can select. NOTE: My Health Food Cookery
Book contains hundreds of tempting and healthful salad sugges-
tions. See the back cover where you may obtain this book.

Many people like to change from the raw vegetable salad to
some kind of fruit salad. This is perfectly all right because a
delicious fruit salad is not only tasty, but it is a real toxic fighter.
Fresh fruits are very aggressive, they will help dissolve and flush
toxic poisons out of the body.

You should eat your fruit salad at the first part of the meal,
as our principle is always to eat something raw at the beginning
of our meals. But when you eat a fruit salad at the beginning
of the meal you should always wait ten minutes before you start
eating your hot food. Fruit leaves the stomach very quickly and
prepares the way for hot food. You may now have two cooked
vegetables—one of them should be of the yellow variety and the

er of the green variety. Your could have a dish of steamed baked carrots and a dish of steamed greens such as spinach, chard, mustard green or turnip greens. These yellow and green vegetables are rich in essential vitamins and minerals.

Again you must control how much of the stimulating foods you are going to add to the diet. That means meat, fish, eggs, cheese and dairy products. Remember, the body requires only a small amount of these foods. No one in the whole wide world can tell you exactly just how much of these foods you can tolerate. If you want to use nuts, seeds and vegetable proteins at this meal, you may do so.

Starch foods such as whole-meal grains and also the protein foods: meats, fish, eggs and dairy products, should be used with great discretion. They are the acid-forming foods and these are the foods that we must use wisely.

For dessert, if you crave a sweet after a meal, you may have fresh baked apples, stewed fruit or occasionally a health pie or cake or cookies made with whole-meal flour and honey. NOTE: My Health Food Cookery Book contains hundreds of health dessert recipes. See the back cover for ordering.

It is best to forget the word sweets and dessert, as it is just another form of over-eating.

LEARN TO SIMPLIFY YOUR DIET

Eating should be one of the greatest joys of life. There is a rule I have followed for many years, and this is, I always get up from the table feeling I could eat just a little more. Remember, you can also over-eat on good food. And remember, the simpler the meal, the better. Most animals live on a mono-diet, that is they eat only one item of food at each meal. And they never suffer from the digestive distress man suffers from. Civilized man seems to want the twelve-course dinner, the buffet dinner, and eats mixture after mixture to abuse his stomach.

Go for simplicity in your eating and you will find the fewer items of food at a meal, the less you are tempted to over-eat. Make the meal a happy occasion, eat by candlelight, play beautiful music on your radio and take your time to chew your food well and, most of all—thoroughly enjoy it. Meal time is no time for serious discussion; it is not a time to argue either. It is an important time in your life for you are building yourself from the food you are eating. Be thankful to God and Nature that you have good natural food to eat. As you eat, millions over the world will go to bed hungry. Malnutrition and starvation are killing thousands this very minute, so be thankful for the food you eat, be thankful that you have been led to a Way of Eating that can keep your body well, strong and youthful!

MY SOUTH SEAS ADVENTURE WITH THE TOXICLESS DIET BODY PURIFICATION AND HEALING SYSTEM

I had been living on the Toxicless Diet Body Purification and Healing System for many years. Through the years I have progressively increased my intake of raw fruits and vegetables and properly cooked fruits and vegetables. I had not eaten breakfast for years.

I had fasted faithfully one twenty-four to thirty-six hour period weekly for many years and had taken many, many fasts of from seven to ten days· some even longer.

Now I was ready to go to the South Sea Islands and see if it was possible to live on a 100% Toxicless Diet, thus a return to the Garden of Eden.

I gave myself a full year to make the experiment. So, I sailed to Tahiti and based myself there. I did visit many Islands of the South Seas, but I never stopped living on the Toxicless· Diet Body Purification and Healing System.

My diet was made exclusively of raw fruit and vegetables, plus properly cooked fruit and vegetables. During this entire year I did not eat fish, flesh of any kind, eggs, grains, or dairy products of any kind. I did from time to time though, eat some nuts and seeds, especially when I took long trips—paddling the heavy out-rigger canoe or climbing mountains.

I exposed my body to the rays of the sunshine all day long. I was on lonely deserted South Sea beaches where I could live absolutely nude as Adam and Eve did in the Garden of Eden.

With the pure, clean Toxicless Diet and the warm tropical sun, I became one with the South Sea Natives. In fact, when people did see me, they would never believe when looking at me that I belonged to the caucasian race. My skin tone and muscle tone was absolutely without a flaw. My strength, endurance, vitality, energy and vigorousness were supreme.

Never before had I attained the physical and internal perfection that I reached on that South Sea Adventure.

Many people who have heard about my South Sea Adventure with the Toxicless Diet Body Purification and Healing System, have asked me the question "Why, if you attained physical perfection, did you return to dirty civilization?"

Open thou mine eyes, that I may behold wondrous things out of thy law.
—Psalm 119:18

FOUND—TRUE SECRET OF HEALTH

My only answer is this, I had made a great discovery and that I could not stay in the South Sea Islands and keep silent. I felt I had to share my discovery with my fellow men. I felt that now I had definitely proved, man can attain the highest state of physical perfection, and I would have been most selfish not to share it with others.

You cannot be selfish and hold on to a great discovery, you must share it, you must teach it. It is by teaching it, that you, the teacher, comes to know his subject better. I knew that I had been privileged to put an entire year in the Garden of Eden. Now, knowing that few people could visit the South Seas like I did, I resolved to help others over the world make their Garden of Eden wherever they were.

In the South Sea Islands the tropical fruits were abundant; the bananas, the papaya, the passion fruit, the coconut and the hundreds of other tropical fruits. It was easy to grow many different vegetables, especially the great vegetable of the South Sea Islands—Taro—a perfect food.

Since I returned from my adventure in the South Seas, I have travelled in many lands, in all kinds of climates, tropical, cold and medium, but I always make it my Garden of Eden. In very cold countries I add more natural starch to my diet, such as whole-meal bread, natural brown rice, whole-meal cereals, and products made from whole-meal grains. I use more nuts and seeds and nut butters, sunflower and sesame seeds. I may even add a few eggs or fish, but I do not care for flesh foods; I never did. You see I was reared on a big farm where I saw blood and slaughter from an early age; we had a big slaughter-house.

There have been times when I have eaten meat. I did research among the Eskimos in the far Arctic Circle and if I had not eaten meat I would not be writing this book today.

Then again I studied the Laplander who lives exclusively on reindeer meat. Again, if I had not eaten reindeer meat I would have starved.

BRAGG DIET GIVES GO-POWER AND HAPPINESS

I enjoy my clean diet of raw fruits and vegetables and properly cooked fruits and vegetables. I have whole-meal products when I feel I need them and raw wheat germ, nuts and nut butters and seeds and seed butter. I thrive on this natural diet, I feel energetic and happy. I am not dogmatic, if I felt that my body needed a piece of flesh I would most assuredly eat it. At times when I can buy some freshly caught fish, I will enjoy it. The South Sea Islanders I met when I was roaming the South Seas ate fish, they even ate raw fish.

After all, there are no two people alike chemically. That is the reason I must, in presenting this Toxicless Diet Body Purification and Healing System, give you the fundamentals of the diet. You must choose your foods.

I have made you aware that the more fruit and vegetables both cooked and raw, you are able to assimilate, the more pure your blood stream and body will be. But you must decide just how much of the flesh, eggs, fish and dairy products you will need. After all, you want a Painless—Tireless—Ageless Body. You know the more toxins you keep out of your body, the healthier and more youthful you will be.

You have made the greatest step towards health and long life when you discard all the devitalized, refined and processed foods of civilization. That alone will put you in a fine nutritional condition.

Now as you add more raw fruit and vegetables to your diet, the cleaner and healthier your body will become.

HAVE SPECIAL HEALTH DAYS

I have what I call my "Special Health Days". On these days I eat only fresh fruit and the juice of fresh fruit. When the watermelons are blood-red, ripe and plentiful, I often have a day or two of only watermelon and watermelon juice. I enjoy going to some beach, lake, river or mountain resort and I take plenty of watermelons, and I feast from one to three days on absolutely nothing but watermelon. I take a large piece of clean cheese cloth and cut my watermelon up and then squeeze the juice. I put it in a glass bottle in the refrigerator and when I am thirsty from playing in the warm sunshine, I drink my fill of watermelon juice.

I have had a full day of fresh black cherries or ripe apricots, and I have even gone a week on nothing but fresh grapes. I often in my very busy life skip a main meal and make it a strictly fruit meal. I seem to work and play harder on a fruit meal.

Of course the heavy meat, ham, egg, refined starch eater would get sick and feel faint on an exclusively fruit meal, let alone a full day of fruit. The person filled with over-flowing toxic poisons must have his white bread, his fried potatoes and his meat with plenty of salt. Then he must wash all this down with some dead beverage like beer, wine, cola drinks, tea or coffee. The toxic persons crave the heavy foods. They love gravies, pies, thick stews, rich heavy sugary desserts, jam, jellies and ice cream.

If they stop eating their rich, heavy diet and eat salads, vegetables and fruits . . . then the body toxins start to flush out of the body, thus giving them a healing crisis. This alarms them, thus if they are weak in character and lack will power to follow this health programme . . . they will go back on their wrong diet. Though I hope all reading this book will be strong and follow this health programme—so they can also experience the wonderful health and vitality I have at eighty-six years young.

When the body is clean and purified you no longer crave the rich heavy foods of civilization.

When you re-educate the 260 taste buds of the mouth, it is almost impossible to let the toxic food enter your system. The clean, re-educated taste buds absolutely refuse to let food trash pass by them. They become the guards to your Holy Temple— The Body.

QUESTIONS MOST ASKED ABOUT THE TOXICLESS DIET BODY PURIFICATION AND HEALING SYSTEM

I travel all over the world giving this Special Programme of Eating. I continually tell students this System is not a set of diets for special named ailments. This System only recognizes one cause of human suffering and that is clogging of the pipes and organs of the human body by toxic materials that have buried themselves into the tissues.

I am not in the curing business. I know of no cures—except the ones the body's internal basic biological functions perform themselves—Nature does all the curing. The body is self-healing and self-repairing. Give the body the right natural chemicals and the body will CURE ITSELF.

Assist nature in her purification and nature will banish your physical problem. This System is not interested in the name of an ailment.

I am only interested in what kind of wrong food and beverages you have used and how long you have used them. If you have been saturating your tissues with toxic poisons for many years, you have built up large amounts of this deadly poison that puts pressure on the nerves. It causes many aches and pains.

When students ask me what they should do for a special ailment, I must give but one answer, and that is to follow the entire System of Toxicless Cleansing. So many people seem to think they should have a special diet for their special physical problem. This is not true. This is not a cure. When the body releases the toxic poisons and the body is again purified there is no longer any distress.

QUESTION: I have suffered from an inflamed colon for years. Raw fruit and vegetables give me terrible pains when I eat them. How can I go on this diet?

ANSWER: Of course you cannot eat a lot of coarse raw fruit and vegetables at once. You will have to start your programme by using soft mashed cooked vegetables, stewed fruit, such as apple sauce, and then gradually add some soft young fresh lettuce to the diet. Then a slice of peeled tomato. Your one day a week fast will help your inflamed colon. No food will pass through your digestive tract for twenty-four hours and this will give the Vital Force a chance to do its healing work. It took you a long, long time to get into this miserable condition and you must be patient and give nature a chance to heal this raw, inflamed digestive tract. Then you should have a day where you eat nothing but apple sauce for twenty-four hours.

QUESTION: Can a child, say five years old, go on the diet?

ANSWER: Yes, in a modified way. A five-year-old child is a growing human and therefore must be given the foods of growth, such as eggs, soy or goat's milk, and natural cheese. Along with these foods teach the child to enjoy fruits, raw and cooked, and raw vegetable salads. The child of five should have whole-meal breads and cereals. Nut butters, peanut butter, etc., are perfect foods for the growing child, so is raw wheat germ and honey. A child can easily fast one twenty-four-hour period weekly. My children fasted one day a week from three years on.

QUESTION: Can a man who does hard physical labour live on the Toxicless Diet Body Purification and Healing System and still keep up his strength?

ANSWER: Eating heavy food does not produce physical strength. This is an old fairy tale that seems to go on and on. Many of my students do the hardest physical labour and yet they live on a balanced diet. They have no breakfast, they may take several whole-meal sandwiches for lunch, along with nuts, seeds and raw vegetables and fruit. Many take a lunch of salads and dried fruits and nuts. Some take a container of salad and a hard-boiled egg. I have tested myself with the hardest physical labour and outside of a few more nuts and sunflower seeds, I can work twelve hours and feel peppy at the end. It's a clean body that has strength and energy. Not one stuffed with heavy foods. I climb high mountains on dried fruits and nuts.

QUESTION: My children will not eat raw fruit or raw vegetables nor will they eat properly cooked vegetables. All they want is meat, fried potatoes, white bread and sweets (candy, cakes, cookies, ice cream and cola soft drinks). What should I do ?

ANSWER: It is too bad that these children did not have a better start nutritionally. Their 260 taste buds are perverted. They crave stimulating foods: protein, starch, fat and refined sugar products. You, as a parent, will have to take control of the situation and you will have to give the orders. Keep the cola drinks, white bread, fried potatoes and the deadly refined sweets out of the house. Prepare a health meal and if they refuse it, that's wonderful—let them fast! Keep them home and confined until they do eat natural foods. Children need strict discipline in their eating. When they develop a real natural hunger they will discover the goodness of a natural diet. Children three years of age and on should also have a twenty-four-hour fast weekly. After they fast, they will relish the salads and natural foods you put before them. They can have a certain amount of meat or fish along with their salad and cooked vegetables. But have them eat the salad first before you give them the cooked foods.

It's your adult, mature mind over your children's mind. You can adjust and control the eating habits of your family. Remember, the Mother prepares with her two hands for her family, either Health or Sickness—Make your choice!

QUESTION: When I eat raw fruit and vegetables, they blow me up with gas. I belch and pass a lot of wind. Also onions, green peppers and cucumbers blow me up. Why is this?

ANSWER: That shows you are loaded with toxic poisons and when these cleansing aggressive foods get into your digestive tract, they really start to clean house. Your weekly twenty-four-hour fast, your "no breakfast" plan and your clean, balanced natural diet will fade this condition away. Keep at it, for this diet is cleaning house.

QUESTION: I do not seem to digest raw fruits and vegetables. They pass out of my body just as I ate them. Why?

ANSWER: You have a crippled digestive tract. Your twenty-four-hour fast weekly and periodically a fast of three days would be helpful to help restore the digestive juices to your digestive tract. Your digestive system has been badly overworked over the years. The tea, coffee, sugar, starch and acid diet have weakened it. Now it will take time to restore the digestive enzymes and other digestive juices so that you can handle these important health foods. Be patient—it takes time to rebuild the digestive system to normal again.

QUESTION: Is it harmful to eat a good meal and then go to bed?

ANSWER: Children eat a hearty meal and go to bed. Animals eat and then sleep. Your food digests whether you are asleep or awake. Now, if you are able to have your main meal during the day—this does break up your day into two days—by giving you a rest period after your main meal—and if you can, by all means take a nap—then you will awake, fresh as a daisy and ready for the rest of the day and evening. So you must adjust to what is best for you and your time. I often have to have my main meal late—but I prefer it in the middle of the day when possible.

QUESTION: I have tried to fast for twenty-four-hours, but I get so weak I cannot stay on my fast. I get violent headaches and get deathly sick in the stomach.

ANSWER: This should definitely convince you what a tremendous amount of toxic poisons you have stored in the pipes, organs and tissues of your body. You had better go to bed during your first few fasts and give your body complete rest and quiet during the fasting. This rest will aid nature in removing the toxic poisons out of your body. Also remember when you get sick to your stomach and feel like throwing up—
—drink water and do so, you must not fight it—please yield! This is usually a sign you have bile and other acids in your system that wish to be removed—thus you get the signal . . . the feeling of sickness in your stomach. You will feel relieved in a matter of minutes, usually after doing so.

QUESTION: When I fast twenty-four hours from dinner to dinner or breakfast to breakfast, the time goes fast—BUT on a three-day fast may I have some Herb Teas to warm and console my stomach?

ANSWER: YES—Herb Teas, like Peppermint, Alfalfa, Chamomile and Anise are refreshing health beverages and permissible when you feel you need something warm in your stomach. You may add a small amount of honey to sweeten if desired. (Remember, China Tea is not part of your health diet—it contains tannic acid which is ideal for uses like hardening shoe leather, etc.—so from now on substitute Herb Teas.)

Also, when fasting you may add the juice of half a small lemon to a glass of water and sweeten with honey if desired. Many people feel this helps them with their fasting and then again others prefer only water. YOU must discover what is best for you!

QUESTION: My children suffer with frequent colds and heavy mucus, will this twenty-four-hour fast weekly help them?

ANSWER: YES—the whole Health Programme will help to make them more alert, vital and healthy. But a factor to consider is maybe your children cannot handle cows' milk and its by-products, for they are heavy mucus formers for people of all ages.

You may substitute Soya powder milk instead of cows' milk. Soya powder milk is even a richer source of protein and other nutrients than cows' milk. You can also use Soya powder milk in your cooking where it calls for cows' milk.

WITH A CLEAN TOXIC-FREE BLOODSTREAM & BODY YOU CAN REACH MENTAL & SPIRITUAL HEIGHTS THAT YOU NEVER DREAMED YOU COULD ACHIEVE

Man is a trinity, he is made of the Physical, Mental and the Spiritual. There is no use trying to reach the heights in the mental and spiritual life when the physical body is decaying. The ancient Greeks finalized man in perfection as having a strong mind in a strong body.

Today millions of people study the Bible daily and benefit from a higher spiritual level. They are truth seekers, they are reaching out for a better way of life, but they are going about it the wrong way. Before you can become an advanced student in spiritual and mental philosophy your body must be clean and free of deadly toxic poisons.

The great spiritual teachers and philosophers have for over 7,000 years recognized the miraculous cleansing power of fasting. Especially our Lord Jesus showed us the importance of fasting and prayer throughout the bible for a closer spiritual walk with him. Buddha, Mohammed and many other spiritual leaders also recognized that fasting was the path to higher spiritual, mental and physical advancements.

When I went into this work many years ago I had only one goal in mind; I wanted to be well, I wanted to stay well and I wanted to be healthy regardless of my calendar years. In other words, I wanted a strong, healthy body with plenty of strength, endurance, vitality and energy.

I attained these goals, but I realized that the Toxicless Diet Body Purification and Healing System was opening other channels of thought to me. I found myself searching for spiritual truth. I questioned the religion of my youth. My mental energy was so high that I was able to do a prodigious amount of reading and study. I searched out brilliant teachers in religion and philosophy and before I knew it, I was attaining a serenity, a tranquillity and peace of mind I had never before experienced. My whole personality was undergoing a change. I no longer worried and fretted over my problems, in fact I liked the challenge that problems presented to me, because I had the mental and spiritual capacity to objectively look at these problems and find the proper solution.

A NEW LIFE FILLS ME WITH JOY

I found myself a happier person—I found that little things could make me laugh and fill me with joy—I discovered the beauty of the stars at night and of the sky during the day—I enjoyed the rain, the wind, and I soon became one with nature! Since my childhood I had carried many fears and anxieties and now I found that these were not true problems and they faded as the night fades in the early morning dawn. I seemed to have been led from the darkness to the light, from the unreal to the real. With fears and anxieties out of my conscience, I was ready to do bigger things in my profession. I had no fears of travelling any place in the world and delivering my message— I found I made friends all over the world—all this I owe to my spiritual and mental growth and body purification.

I have found that I am gradually developing extra sensory perception. I have learned to concentrate in my meditations and use this extra sensory perception to solve future conditions that I must face. I have found answers that have saved me many hours of anxiety and worry.

Many people talk about relaxing—I used to talk about relaxing—but it was only after years of consistent fasting and purification through diet, that I really learned to relax. Each day of my life, I am able to release all the tensions from my nerves and muscles and revive my vitality and energy through complete relaxation. I sleep better now, than I did when I was a child I find that no matter where I am, no matter what the noise or excitement may be, I can sit or lie down, close my eyes and completely relax.

I find that I am able to understand other people better when they become angry and emotional, and therefore I am able to help them calm themselves.

I feel I am growing, not only on the physical side, I feel that I am not only building a powerful physical body, but I believe, through the Cleansing Programme, I am advancing on the Mental and the Spiritual side. I constantly search for light and truth and education along all lines. I find that I have great interest in everything that is happening in the world. I find I understand people better and in understanding others, I am able to better understand myself.

This way of life opens many doors, and these doors all lead to the higher life, and after all, as we journey through life we should grow Physically, Mentally and Spiritually. Hundreds of my students write and tell me of this newly discovered strength in Mental and Spiritual Strength growth they are experiencing. They rejoice when they have found Peace of Mind and the true Joy of Living.

I am a happy man, I have no worries, no fears and no false ambitions. I lead a simple, happy life and I owe it all to the fact that as my body gets cleaner, I advance on all planes of living—the Physical, the Mental and the Spiritual.

THE IMPORTANCE OF SUNBATHING

I believe this is absolutely essential—that everyone should take every opportunity they can, to expose their body to the life-giving rays of sunshine. I believe that every person must understand the pigment of their skin and not overdo exposure to the rays of the sun.

I believe that the alpine sunshine, at an altitude of 5,000 feet in the Swiss Alps, played a tremendous part in my recovery from tuberculosis. When I arrived at Dr. Rollier's Sanatorium, my introduction to sunbathing was supervised closely. The first day in the alpine sun I only exposed my feet, and each day the Doctor instructed me to expose more of my body to the direct rays of the sun. My conditioning period to expose my whole body to the sunshine extended over a period of three months—by that time my body was conditioned to take hours of sunshine. The Doctor believed that the best rays of the sun were in the early morning rays and in the late afternoon rays. I would start my sunbathing programme as early as 6 a.m. when the first rays of the sun appeared. In the cool of the morning the ultra-violet rays, which are the healing rays, are at their highest point of radiation. By 11 a.m. the ultra-violet rays start to disappear and the hot infra-red rays take over. That was the time the Doctor advised his patients to come out of the sun. Then again after 3 p.m. we were allowed to expose our body to the ultra-violet rays that had now appeared, as the hot infra-red rays had gone.

USE CAUTION WHEN SUNBATHING

I believe many people damage their skin by too long exposure to the hot infra-red rays. Most people are looking for a tan, so they smear a lot of grease over themselves and expose themselves to the burning rays, which I have explained to you are the infra-red rays. There is no doubt about it—serious damage is done to the skin by unscientific sunbathing.

Most people have so much toxic acid in their skin, that when the rays of sunshine strike these surface toxins, severe damage can be done to the skin. Sunbathing should be done slowly, so that there is no violent reaction on the skin, and this means that the time to sunbathe is from sunrise to 11 a.m. and from 3 p.m. until sundown. You will find as you detoxicate your body and eliminate toxic acids, you will be able to develop a beautiful natural tan. Most people are so full of toxic acid that when they go out into the sunshine all they get is severe sunburn. Sunburn can even cause death—the sun's rays are powerful and while we can use them judiciously, we should always use them with great caution. Very fair people should do all their sunbathing in the early rays of the morning and in the late afternoon.

DOCTOR SUNSHINE

Doctor Sunshine's speciality is heliotheraphy, and his great prescription is solar energy. Each tiny blade of grass, every vine, tree, bush, flower, fruit, and vegetable draws its life from solar energy. All living things on earth depend on solar energy for their very existence. This earth would be a barren, frigid place if it were not for the magic rays of the sun. The sun gives us light, and were it not for LIGHT, there would be No You or Me.

The person who is starved of the vital rays of the sun has a half-dead look. He is actually dying for the want of solar energy. Weak, ailing, anemic people are all sun-starved, and in my opinion, many people are sick simply because they too are starving for sunshine.

SUNSHINE—THE HEALER

The rays of the sun are powerful germicides. As the skin imbibes more of these rays, it stores up enormous amounts of this germ-killing energy. The sun provides one of the finest remedies for the nervous person, who is filled with anxiety, worry, frustration, stresses, and strains. When these tense people lie in the sunshine, its powerful rays give them what the nerves and body are crying out for, and that is relaxation. Sunshine is a tonic, a stimulant and, above all, the GREAT HEALER ! As you bask in the warm sunshine, millions of nerve endings absorb the solar energy and transform it to the nervous system of the body.

Make this experiment, determine the value of sunshine in the matter of life and death. Find a beautiful lawn, where the grass is like a green carpet . . . Cover up a small space of that beautiful lawn with a small piece of wood or a piece of metal. Day by day you will notice that the beautiful grass that is full of plant blood, Chlorophyll, will start to fade and turns a sickly yellow. Then the tragedy happens—it withers and dies—death by sun starvation.

EAT SUN-COOKED FOODS

The same thing happens in your body without the life-giving rays of the sun, and when you fail to eat an abundance of sun-cooked foods such as ripe fruits, and vegetables.

We must have the direct rays of the sun on our bodies and we must eat at least fifty per cent of food that has been ripened by the sun's rays. When we eat fresh fruits and vegetables, we absorb blood of the plant, the rich, nourishing Chlorophyll. Chlorophyll is the solar energy that the plant has absorbed from the sun, the richest and most nourishing food you can put into your body. **" Chlorophyll is liquid sunshine."** Green plants alone possess the secret of how to capture this powerful solar energy and pass it on to man and every other living creature. When you put sunshine on the outside of your body, and eat fifty per cent raw fruits and vegetables in your daily diet, you are going to fairly glow with radiant health.

We are children of the sunshine, our life depends upon the sun to produce our food and we can contribute to our bank of health by taking sunbaths. If you cannot take a sunbath, then you should at least take an airbath. In the privacy of your own room you can open the windows and allow the fresh air to

stimulate the skin of your body—sunbaths and airbaths are extra
ways that you can add more vitality to your body.

THE IMPORTANCE OF EXERCISE

You have six hundred and thirty-three muscles, and these
muscles must all be used. If you do not use them, you lose
them, if they are not used they lose their tone, their strength and
their flexibility. Exercise need not be violent and there are
hundreds of ways to exercise the human body. Best and greatest
of all exercise is walking and no special equipment is required
except a good pair of shoes. You can make your walk vigorous
or you can take it easy. When you walk and breathe in deeply
as you stride along you are building vital power. After walking,
I would say that swimming is the second greatest exercise. Sports
of any kind that bring into play the muscles of the body should
be part of your daily health programme. Tennis, even gardening,
can be considered wonderful exercise. Then you should have
a twenty-minute programme of general physical fitness exercises.

The best exercise for the lower abdomen and lower back
muscles is to lie on your back and raise both your legs up slowly
—then slowly lower them until your heels almost touch the
floor, then slowly raise back up to a vertical position again.
Important—do this exercise slowly and increase the repetitions
daily until you can do thirty. This exercise is good for the
internal and external abdomen muscles—The Setup Exercise:
Lie flat on your back with your arms extended backward over
your head, now come up to a sitting position and touch your toes.
Slowly lower your body back to the prone position. Repeat this
exercise daily until in time you can do with ease twenty repetitions.

Also for relieving swollen ankles and feet—if you will lie on
the bed or floor and place your feet up on the wall, pushing your
buttocks as close to the wall as possible—this will bring soothing
relief to your legs and ankles; ten—twenty minutes is ideal while
you are reading your paper or book or napping.

Because men or women are athletic and powerfully built with
great strength and endurance, that does not mean that they are
internally clean. Far from it. Many athletic people over-eat on
the heavy, stimulating foods. I know weightlifters who eat four
or five pounds of meat daily, drink quarts of milk and stuff other
heavy stimulating foods into their stomachs. It gives them big,
powerful muscles and great physical powers, but I have seen
many of those former athletes die in their early fifties and sixties.
No, athletes do not live longer than others. When they stop

their heavy exercising and thus slow down their circulation, the toxic poisons build up from the high protein and stimulating diet. The toxic poisons are now not being flushed out by the heavy exercising which they stopped—THEN they start to suffer with the same ailments that the non-athletic person suffers with.

It is not only muscle, or physical fitness that counts, it all comes down to the basic point " HOW CLEAN ARE YOU INTERNALLY?"

DAILY EXERCISE A MUST

I am 100% for physical fitness and exercise! Now, please do not misunderstand me. I think the ideal combination of natural nutrition and exercise can accomplish wonders for a person. I love hiking, swimming, tennis, mountain climbing, progressive weight-training. I am an active man. I look forward every day of my life to my physical activity. To over-rest is to rust. If you don't use your muscles—your muscles will lose their firmness, tone and their strength. But I also know I **must** keep my body clean of toxic poisons by consistent eating of raw fruit and vegetables and by the weekly twenty-four-hour fast, plus three or four times a year, a fast from seven to ten days.

When you follow a Health Programme like this, you are filled with inexhaustible vitality and energy. You are like a child who is healthy, you become an active, happy person. You love life and activity . . . walking, swimming, and keeping active regardless of your calendar years. NOTE: My book "The Golden Keys to Internal Physical Fitness" goes deeply into the Science of Corrective, Health Building Exercises. You will find where you may obtain this book on the back cover.

THE IMPORTANCE OF DEEP BREATHING FOR OXYGEN IS OUR INVISIBLE FOOD

We are breathing machines and must have oxygen constantly or we will perish. The more oxygen we can get into the system, the cleaner our bodies are going to be, and by cleaning the body we are able to absorb more life-giving oxygen into the tissues. I want you to know we are air-gas machines, we live at the bottom of a sea of oxygen—the atmosphere extends seventy miles above us and has a pressure of fourteen pounds per square inch. The latin word " spira " means oxygen, air and then spirit, the breath of God is in fact oxygen and therefore air.

He who cannot find time for exercise, will have to find time for illness.

—Lord Derby

Most people are shallow breathers, they only get oxygen in the upper regions of the lungs instead of the deep lower regions of the lungs. They become oxygen starved, pale and sallow looking.

DIRECTIONS FOR FILLING THE ENTIRE LUNGS WITH LIFE-GIVING OXYGEN

Lie flat on your back, either in bed or on the floor, then slowly inhale through your nose, but in inhaling do not move the upper chest or the abdominal region, take in a long slow breath—while you are doing this, place your hands on the lower ribs, which are known as the floating ribs. NOW, if you are breathing correctly you can feel the lower ribs expand. Take in a full, long breath; when you feel that your lungs are filled to capacity with air, expel the breath with a long open-mouth sigh. In this way you will completely clean the lungs of the carbon dioxide which must be expelled, as this is the most deadly poison our body creates. After you have expelled the breath, with this long open-mouth sigh, hold the breath for a full ten seconds, then repeat the same routine, long slow breath inhaled, filling the lower lungs and expanding the lower floating ribs, then expel the air with an open-mouth sigh, then hold the breath for ten seconds, then repeat. This should be done twice a day, on arising and on retiring. Do this breathing exercise fifteen times, morning and night.

During the waking hours, every time you can think about it, take several of these long deep breaths. NOTE: My book, "Bragg System of Super Brain Breathing", can give you a marvellous technique of driving oxygen and air into any part of the body; into the brain, sinus cavities, ears, nose and throat.

Breathing is the most important function in raising the body's vitality to its highest potential. It is true that by deep breathing you do remove toxic poisons by higher air pressure and counter pressure in this way. It is true that you can remove and eliminate encumbrances of foreign matter by long, full, deep breaths. The body has a great capacity for oxygen and you should constantly keep this in mind, because the more air you get in the body the more toxic poisons you are going to burn up, and the more vitality you are going to create. In other words, the problem of creating more energy and better body functioning, consists in unobstructed perfect circulation by air pressure, and in a vital elasticity of the tissues through correct foods; this is the necessary counter pressure for the functions of life. So you see, oxygen is a detoxifier. It is like fasting . . . it helps to remove poisons from the body. The cleaner your body becomes through fasting, and a preponderance of raw fruits and vegetables, the more your energy will increase by many, many times. With a clean, purified body and an abundance of oxygen, you can have a youthful and healthful condition, and maintain this high state of physical efficiency for an indefinite number of years.

YOUR TONGUE NEVER LIES

The tongue should be called " The Magic Mirror ". The tongue reveals the great amount of toxic poison that is stored in the body.

One of the means a doctor uses to diagnose a person is to say, " Let me see your tongue ". When the doctor sees a white-coated tongue, he knows that person is in a highly toxic condition. This is one of the oldest methods of diagnosis of man.

Remember, the tongue is one end of a tube that is thirty feet long, it extends from your mouth to the anus. When the tongue is coated it shows that nature is trying to simulate some of the deep buried toxins of the body.

Sick people have heavily-coated tongues and with it a bad breath. Now, when you fast a few days or go on a strict fruit diet such as apples or oranges you will at once notice that the tongue will become heavily coated. The fasting and the strict diet starts to loosen the filthy toxic poisons of the body. The tongue is " the Magic Mirror " not only of the stomach, but the entire mucus membrane system, as well. You can gargle a solution of half fresh lemon juice and half water and then scrape your tongue with a spoon and that spoon will show you the toxic slime that is on the tongue. You can do this three or four times a day during a complete water fast or fruit diet and you will still get plenty of this toxic slime off the tongue. It is an accurate indication of the amount of decaying filth,   rotting mucus and other toxic poisons accumulated in the tissues of your entire body, now being eliminated on the inside surface of the stomach, intestines and from every vital organ of the body. You may also use as a gargle one tablespoon of cider vinegar to a glass of water as an aid in removing mucus from the throat area. This also gives relief from a sore throat or cold.

You can now see by the coated tongue how much toxic poison you have stored in your body. The tongue's surface reveals to the person the great amount of encumbrance that has been clogging up the entire body since childhood, through wrong, toxic-forming foods.

That is the reason I am not interested in the name of your physical trouble. All physical problems are due to a local clogging of the circulation, tissues, and the entire pipe system.

If you have a pain in your shoulder and it is inflamed, it could be given the name, bursitis. But I see it only as concentrated toxic poisons at that point. The pain and inflammation are caused from too heavy a concentration of toxic poisons in the shoulder. Naturally, there will be inflammation caused by friction and heavy congestion.

When a person with this condition fasts, the tongue will take on a heavy white coating, showing that the body, as soon as a person stops eating, will start eliminating the toxic poisons. In a few days of strict water fasting, you will get some relief from the pain in your shoulder—depending on the intensity of the condition.

THE HUMAN PIPE SYSTEM MUST BE
KEPT CLEAN

Let me repeat, every physical problem a person suffers with is constitutional clogging. The entire human pipe system, especially the microscopically small capillaries (the smallest pipes in the body, about the size of a human hair), are "chronically" clogged, through the foodless foods of civilization.

There are no special diets that can clean a dirty, heavily-coated tongue. This is the reason I give no special diets for special ailments. This is the reason that I do not believe in "cures" of any kind.

To be well, and to stay well and free from aches and pains, you must live each day so that you eliminate the toxic poisons you have accumulated over the years, and to so eat that you build no more toxic poisons in the body.

The Toxicless Diet Body Purification and Healing System calls for large amounts of fresh vegetables and fruits and properly cooked vegetables; weekly fasts of twenty-four hours and periodic fasts of from seven to ten days. I know what this System of Internal Purification can do for the sick and prematurely old person. For over seventy years I have been using this System on myself and thousands of my students all over the world. I have received thousands of letters from grateful students who have put this System to the test and it worked for them . . . when every other method failed, this System was successful.

55

The success of this System is that it works on the person to improve the whole body and not the symptom. I am NOT interested in symptoms. I am NOT interested in the name of a bad place in the body. I am interested in just one thing . . .

"CLEAN THOSE FILTHY TOXIC POISONS OUT OF THE BODY"

The characteristics of tissue construction, especially of the important internal organs, such as the liver, kidneys, lungs and glands, are all very much like those of a sponge. Now I want you to imagine a sponge soaked with a sticky glue or paste. As a person lives on the foodless foods of civilization, the vital organs begin to fill up with this slimy paste or glue (toxic poisons). No wonder they die of horrible diseases of the liver, kidneys and lungs. They actually become so clogged with these slimy, sticky, decaying toxic poisons that the vital organ can no longer function.

Death by toxic poisoning. Death by clogging of the entire pipe system. Now, do you know why I want you to detoxicate? . . . to cleanse and purify your body? It is the only natural way to CURE YOURSELF!

FASTING—NATURE'S MASTER HEALER

Nature heals through—FASTING—every physical problem that it is possible to heal. This alone definitely proves that Mother Nature recognizes but one problem, and that in every body the largest factors are always toxic poisons, decaying mucus, foreign matter, Uric acid, pus and many other toxic poisons.

Just look what happens to people when they suffer from a common cold. They run a high fever, they eliminate great masses of mucus and phlegm from the sinus cavities of the head, from the throat, lungs and bronchial tubes. A common cold is the body's way of saying "I must get rid of this toxic slime to survive". And a healing crisis is started by the Vital Force of the body.

The average person who experiences a cold takes absolutely no blame for this condition. Oh, no, they will say "I got my feet wet and caught a cold". "I sat in a draught and caught a cold." Or "I caught the cold from a bug my brother brought home from school" . . . Excuses, excuses! Never placing the blame exactly on themselves. Three times a day at meals these people load the mucus-forming foods into their bodies. They eat ice cream, cakes, candy, soft drinks, tea and coffee filled with

---

The elimination of waste products by Fasting increases longevity.
—Alexis Carrel, M.D., Famous Scientist

refined white sugar, and when this mess decays in their bodies they cry out, "I caught this cold, poor me". Yes, poor ignorant you. Ignorance is bliss.

You do not catch colds, you develop colds from your rotten one-sided, dead diet.

URINE REVEALS THE AMOUNT OF TOXIC POISONS IN THE BODY

The urine tells the story of the amount of toxic poisons in the body.

All you have to do is start a strict water fast (nothing else but water). And during the days you fast, drink plenty of water. Now, the first thing in the morning take a bottle and secure a specimen of your urine. Seal the top of this bottle so no air can get in. Take a piece of tape and write the date you took the specimen of urine. Now write the day of the fast. Let's say you are going to take a seven-day fast. Each morning you take your specimen and you put it away in a closet and let it cool and settle.

As it cools and settles you get a revelation before your very eyes. After a week you see the big clouds of slimy putrid mucus. Then as the days pass, even weeks and months, right there before your very eyes you see the horrible, decaying filth that you eliminated during your fast. It has weight. It had burdened your vital organs.

I have fasted thousands in my long career and I have saved many bottles of urine from my fasters. If you looked at them you would hardly believe your eyes. But there they are, showing what filth humans carry around with them.

And sometimes I meet some boastful ass who will say, " I eat anything, and I am strong and healthy ". I simply reply " You are a walking manure pile ". " Just let me fast you for a week to ten days and I will have you on the flat of your back, stewing in your own decaying, toxic poisons."

As I have told you, physical strength, athletic ability and physical fitness have nothing to do with health. The stronger they are, the harder they fall when the body clogs up with decaying toxic poisons.

INFECTIONS, GERMS, BUGS, VIRUS AND BACTERIA ARE SCAVENGERS

You often hear people say " A new virus is attacking people. It seems that everyone is picking it up." That is exactly right, there are thousands of germs floating around everywhere, and remember they are here for a purpose. They are scavengers, they clean up decaying filth. If that decaying filth happens to be in your body, they are going to start eating that toxic slime.

Just remember it is impossible for any kind of germ or virus to attack clean, healthy tissue. They only eat decaying toxic matter. Personally, I have no fear of infection from any germ or bug. I fast, I eat plenty of raw fruit and raw vegetables, and properly cooked fruits and vegetables. I am very jealous of my body, therefore I do not put the dead food of civilization into my fine body instrument.

Dirty blood picks up infections. Clean blood is your protection against infection.

If by wrong eating you create decaying matter in your body, it is only a part of nature's plan that germs will come and eat this dead substance. Germs never attack clean, toxic-free tissue or clean, toxic-free blood.

As a child, I was fed a terrible diet of refined white flour products, refined white sugar products such as ice cream, cakes, cookies, jams, jellies, candies and many foods that were unwholesome and devitalised. I picked up all the children's diseases: chicken-pox, mumps, whooping cough and many others. Why? Because my diet put dirty, foul toxins in my tissues and blood stream. So, the germs came and had a feast on my internal poisons.

My own children were reared on the Toxicless Diet Body Purification and Healing System, consequently they never suffered from any of the so-called children's diseases.

Infectious diseases kill many humans. The germs attack the body to eat the decaying toxic matter and many times destroy vital organs that cause death. By following this Body Purification Programme YOU can build within your body chemistry a powerful immunity against the attack of germs. Germs eat only decaying matter. Keep clean inside. A powerful, nutritionally fit blood stream is your greatest defence against the invasion of germs. Germs thrive in a dirty blood stream and they perish in a clean one.

BANISH CONSTIPATION—NATURE'S WAY

Constipation is often referred to as the cause of many serious physical problems in the body.

Few people know what normal bowel evacuation means. The average person feels that if they have one bowel evacuation a day they are not constipated. This is not true. People who only have one bowel movement a day are chronically constipated, and carry 5—10 lbs. of putrefying and fermenting food material in the lower bowel. This produces irritation to the delicate lining of the bowel, whereby it either tries to get rid of the irritations quickly, which results in a diarrhoea, or puts a spastic clamp on the intestines to keep them from producing further, resulting in stasis or constipation.

Civilized people never seem to go to the root cause of their constipation—wrong diet and lack of exercise of the internal and the external muscles of the abdomen.

In America alone they spend $368 million a year to try to move the constipated bowels. All civilized countries sell a tremendous amount of laxatives and cathartics, to try to move the constipated bowels. The chief reason we need so much bowel " DYNAMITE " is because we eat so much lifeless, food-less, empty-calorie foods. Our foods have lost their B-complex vitamins, without which we cannot have a healthy, clean intestinal tract. Our digestive tract will lack tone unless vitamin B_1, especially, is present. In addition, our diets consist of too many foods that have been cooked to a soft, mushy consistency, instead of being crisp and chewy; with the lack of tough cellulose fibres of raw vegetables which act as helpful, tiny intestinal brooms, giving mobility, bulk, moisture and lubrication to the colon.

The Toxicless Diet Body Purification and Healing System emphasizes at all times that a person should have one to two raw coarse salads a day, and the base of these salads should be raw chopped or grated cabbage, carrots, beetroot and celery. Cellulose, which is the fleshy part of fresh, uncooked fruits and vegetables, provides a colloidal property which retains water and acts as soft bulk throughout the entire digestive system.

If for any reason you cannot eat rough raw foods, or if you cannot tolerate them, make a flaxseed tea and drink it after each meal. Use one heaped tablespoonful of flaxseed to one cup of water, bring to boil and let it cook with a moderate rolling boil for ten—fifteen minutes. Strain the seeds and drink the thick tea which the flaxseeds will produce.

Another suggestion for the relief of constipation is to one cup of hot water mix one heaped tablespoonful of crude black strap molasses—one on arising, one after the midday meal and one before retiring.

The more natural the food you eat, the more radiant health you will enjoy and you will be better able to promote the higher life of love and brotherhood.
—Patricia Bragg

THE IMPORTANCE OF B-COMPLEX
VITAMINS FOR INTESTINAL HEALTH

The muscles of the intestinal tract may become flabby and prolapsed if the B-complex vitamins, especially B_1 are not in abundance in the diet. These water-soluble vitamins are not stored, but are lost in perspiration and urine, so be sure to include in your diet plenty of foods that are rich in the B vitamins. Here are some of the foods rich in B vitamins: raw wheat germ, brewers yeast, black strap molasses, rice polishings, barley, soya beans, dried peas and beans, peanuts, corn meal, buckwheat groats, mushrooms, broccoli, turnip and mustard greens, spinach, cabbage, peas, cantaloupe, grapefruit and oranges. Also found in fish, beef steak, beef heart, lamb kidney, and egg yolks.

Never, under any circumstances, use mineral oil as a laxative. It robs the body of the fat-soluble vitamins (A, D, E and F) that are waiting to be assimilated in the intestinal tract.

Never use enemas or high colonic irrigations unless in cases of sickness. Your nerves move your bowels and they can and will do the job if your vitamin B-complex intake is adequate, and if your diet is correctly balanced.

You should have a bowel movement on arising and one within an hour after each meal. Out-go must equal intake. Make it a practice to go to the toilet within twenty—thirty minutes after a meal and concentrate your entire mind on having a bowel evacuation. Use a twelve—fourteen inch footstool in front of the toilet to bring your feet up higher, so that the abdominal muscles can contract and relax normally, aiding in a complete bowel movement. You should make a ten-minute effort to move the bowels after each meal. Cleanliness of the colon is important for superior health. If you are made miserable with tenderness, soreness, or hemorrhaging of the rectum, a peeled garlic bud, oiled and inserted as a suppository and allowed to remain overnight has been found most healing.

If your bowel movement is dry, see that your liquid intake is from six—eight glasses in the form of water, vegetable juice or fruit juice. Many people suffer from constipation because they are dehydrated—remember salt, tea, coffee, alcohol, cola drinks and soft drinks are dehydrating. Use of the functions of the lower bowel is to remove surplus water from the waste. If the wastes are not evacuated, and remain in the colon too long, a great deal of water is removed, the stool becomes too hard to eliminate without causing pain or even damage to the delicate membranes.

Remember, there is nothing as important as good elimination in the bowels, so take care of this important function after each meal before too much of the liquid has been absorbed.

Don't tell me you are too busy. Bowel elimination is vital to vigorous health—these poisons must be moved out of the body —no meal should stay in the human's colon more than thirty-six hours. I have so trained my bowels that they move a meal out of my body in sixteen—eighteen hours, and never more than twenty-four hours.

When the normal rhythm of bowel evacuation is reached you are going to find many of your physical problems will vanish.

Keep clean inside, this is the Secret of Health, Youthfulness and Long Life.

MY PERSONAL MESSAGE TO MY STUDENTS

It is my sincere desire that each one of my students attains Paradisaical Health, freedom from every nagging and tormenting human ailment and a " God-like " being.

After intelligent and careful study of the foregoing you must now know that all human physical problems consist of a fermenting and decaying mass of material in the human body, many years old, and it is concentrated in the intestines and colon.

I have taught you that there is no special diet for any special ailment. My System of Internal Purification is one of cleansing by eating more raw fruits and vegetables and fasting. It is only through progressive cleansing that the human " cesspool " can be banished. I have told you that you will go through cleansing crises from time to time—at these times you will become weak and in many instances will become greatly discouraged. This is the time you must have great strength, because it is during these crises, when you feel the worst, that you are doing the greatest amount of cleansing. This is why weaklings, cry-babies and people without intestinal fortitude fail in this perfect System of Regeneration and Rejuvenation.

Weaklings want a cure that requires no effort on their part. Nature does not work that way. The average unfortunate sick person thinks of the Lord as the kind and forgiving Father who will allow him to enter the Garden of Eden effortlessly and unpunished for any violation of his laws in nature.

You can find and live in your Garden of Eden no matter where you live, regardless of the climate; all you have to do is to purify the body of its vile toxic poisons, and you will reach the stage of health and youthfulness that you never ever thought was possible. You can reach a stage of agelessness, where actually the chronological age stands still, and pathological age will make you younger.

When your body is free of deadly toxic material, you will reach the physical, mental and spiritual state that will give you happiness every waking hour and add many youthful, active, joyous years to your life.

To attain this High State of Physical, Mental and Spiritual Health, Your Motto will be " HEALTH FIRST "!

Be so strong Physically, Mentally and Spiritually that nothing can ever bring you back to the wrong way of living.

Make your mind the master of your body.

God bless you, and give you the strength and the courage and the patience to win your battle to re-enter the Garden of Eden.

Yours for Health, Strength, Vitality, Happiness and Long-lasting Youthfulness,

Paul C. Bragg   *Patricia Bragg*

UNCOMPLICATE YOUR LIVING

Living is a continual lesson in problem solving, but the trick is to know where to start. No excuses — start your Health Program Today.

"Living under conditions of modern life, it is important to bear in mind that the perparation and refinement of food products either entirely eliminates or in part destroys the vital elements in the original materials." — **U.S. Dept. of Agriculture**

"Now learn what and how great benefits a temperate diet will bring with it. In the first place, you enjoy good health.
— **Horace, 65-8 B.C.**

Life cannot be maintained unless life be taken in, and this is best done by making at least 60 percent of your diet raw and cooked vegetables, with a plentiful supply of fresh juicy fruits. — **Patricia Bragg**

"Your eyes shall be opened, and ye shall be as gods, knowing good and evil."
—Genesis 3:5

62

WE THANK THEE

For flowers that bloom about our feet;
  For song of bird and hum of bee;
For all things fair we hear or see,
  Father in heaven we thank Thee!
For blue of stream and blue of sky;
  For pleasant shade of branches high;
For fragrant air and cooling breeze;
  For beauty of the blooming trees,
Father in heaven, we thank Thee!
  For mother-love and father-care,
For brothers strong and sisters fair;
  For love at home and here each day;
For guidance lest we go astray,
  Father in heaven, we thank Thee!
For this new morning with its light;
  For rest and shelter of the night;
For health and food, for love and friends;
  For every thing His goodness sends,
Father in heaven, we thank Thee!
                    - Ralph Waldo Emerson

Ponce de Leon,

Searched for the "Fountain of Youth".

If he had only known —

— it's within us...

Created by the food we eat!

"Food can make or break you!"

63

Take time
for **12** things

1 *Take time to Work*—
it is the price of success.

2 *Take time to Think*—
it is the source of power.

3 *Take time to Play*—
it is the secret of youth.

4 *Take time to Read*—
it is the foundation of knowledge.

5 *Take time to Worship*—
it is the highway of reverance and washes the
dust of earth from our eyes.

6 *Take time to Help and Enjoy Friends*—
it is the source of happiness.

7 *Take time to Love*—
it is the one sacrament of life.

8 *Take time to Dream*—
it hitches the soul to the stars.

9 *Take time to Laugh*—
it is the singing that helps with life's loads.

10 *Take time for Beauty*—
it is everywhere in nature.

11 *Take time for Health*—
it is the true wealth and treasure of life.

12 *Take time to Plan*—
it is the secret of being able to have time to
take time for the first eleven things.

BRAGG BLESSINGS

*From the Bragg home to your home we share our years of health
knowledge—years of living close to God and Nature and what joys of
fruitful, radiant living this produces—this my Father and I share
with you and your loved ones.*

With blessings for Health
and Happiness,

Patricia Bragg

LAW OF LIFE

Man's body was created according to the laws of physics and chemistry, which are the Creator's own laws. They never vary. His law is written upon every nerve, every muscle, every faculty, which has been entrusted to us.

These laws govern the cells, tissues, and organs of the body as they carry on their various functions. They operate largely through the complex network of nerves that run throughout the body. They act through the central nervous system, from which nerve impulses originate, and through the autonomic nervous system, that part of the network not under the direct control of the will.

-Henry W. Vollmer, M.D.

PLEASE REMEMBER
YOUR HEALTH IS YOUR WEALTH

Open thou mine eyes, that I may behold wondrous things out of thy law. —Psalm 119:18

Of all the knowledge, that most worth having is knowledge about health. The first requisite of a good life is to be a healthy person. —Herbert Spencer

When you have been stricken by illness, your new car, your new home, your new big bank balance—all these fade into unimportance until you have regained your vigor and zest for living again.
—Peter J. Steincrohn, M.D.

If your food is devitalized, the important elements of nourishment have been removed, or if its value has been diminished by wrong cooking processes—you can then starve to death on a full stomach.

The unexamined life is not worth living. It is a time to re-evaluate your past as a guide to your future. —Socrates

TIME

I have just a little minute,
Only sixty seconds in it,
Just a tiny little minute,
Give account if I abuse it;
Forced upon me; can't refuse it.
Didn't seek it, didn't choose it,
But it's up to me to use it.
I must suffer if I lose it;
But eternity is in it.—Unknown

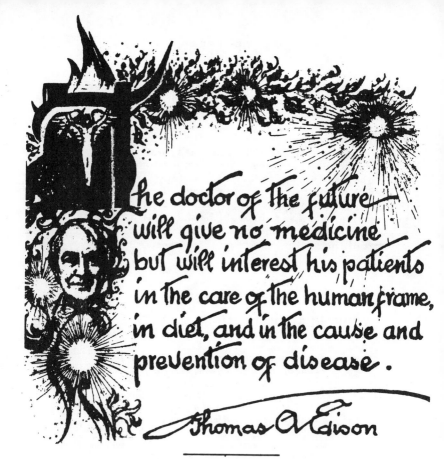

The doctor of the future will give no medicine but will interest his patients in the care of the human frame, in diet, and in the cause and prevention of disease.

Thomas A. Edison

LAW OF LIFE

Man's body was created according to the laws of physics and chemistry, which are the Creator's own laws. They never vary. His law is written upon every nerve, every muscle, every faculty, which has been entrusted to us. These laws govern the cells, tissues, and organs of the body as they carry on their various functions. They operate largely through the complex network of nerves that run throughout the body. They act through the central nervous system, from which nerve impulses originate, and through the autonomic nervous system, that part of the network not under the direct control of the will.   -Henry W. Vollmer, M.D.

Every man is the builder of a temple called his body...We are all sculptors and painters, and our material is our own flesh and blood and bones. Any nobleness begins at once to refine a man's features, any meanness or sensuality to imbrute them.   – Henry David Thoreau

THE TREE OF TOXEMIA

IN THE SOIL OF
HUMAN HABITS AND BEHAVIOR

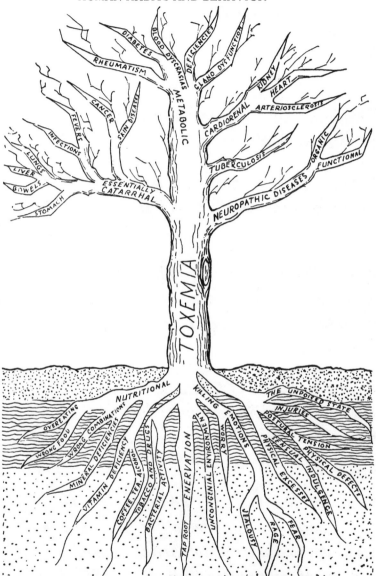

Many people go throughout life committing partial suicide — destroying their health, youth, beauty, talents, energies, creative qualities. Indeed, to learn how to be good to oneself is often more difficult than to learn how to be good to others.

— Paul C. Bragg

Slow Me Down, Lord

Slow me down, Lord

Ease the pounding of my heart by the quieting of my mind.

Steady my hurried pace with a vision of the eternal reach of time.

Give me, amid the confusion of the day, the calmness of the everlasting hills.

Break the tensions of my nerves and muscles with the soothing music of the singing streams that live in my memory. Help me to know the magical, restoring power of sleep.

Teach me the art of taking minute vacations—of slowing down to look at a flower, to chat with a friend, to pat a dog, to read a few lines from a good book.

Slow me down, Lord, and inspire me to send my roots deep into the soil of lifes enduring values that I may grow toward the stars of my greater destiny.

———

Now I see the secret of the making of the best persons, it is to grow in the open air, and eat and sleep with the earth.   -Walt Whitman

HEALTHY HEART HABITS FOR A LONG VITAL LIFE

Remember, you are what you eat, drink & do, so eat a low-fat, low-sugar, high-fiber diet of natural whole grains and starches, fresh salad greens, sprouts, vegetables, fresh fruits, raw seeds, nuts, pure juices and distilled water (chemical free).

Earn your food with daily exercise, for regular exercise improves your health, stamina, flexibility, endurance, & helps open up the cardiovascular system. Only 45 minutes a day can do miracles for your mind and body.

We are made of tubes: to help keep them clean & open, add raw oat bran, 2-3 tablespoons daily to juices, pep drinks, herbal teas, soups, hot cereals, foods, etc. Just be sure that it's wet and expanded for 2 minutes.

Niacin (B-3) helps also to cleanse and open the cardiovascular system. Take regular-released Niacin (100 mg) with one meal daily. After cholesterol level reaches 180 or lower, you can take Niacin once or twice weekly.

Remember, your heart needs a good balance of nutrients, so take a natural vitamin-mineral food supplement with extra vitamin E (mixed Tocopherols), the new Ester-C, Magnesium and Beta Carotene, for these are your heart's super helpers!

Also use this amazing enzyme SOD (super oxide dismutase) for it helps flush out dangerous free radicals that can cause havoc with your cardiovascular pipes and general health. Latest research shows extra benefits...promotes longevity, slows aging & fights arthritis & its stiffness, swelling & pain, and it helps prevent jet lag, exhaustion and cataracts.

Count your blessings daily while you do your brisk walking and exercises with these affirmations – "health! strength! youth! vitality! peace! laughter! humbleness! energy! understanding! forgiveness! joy! and love!"– and soon all these qualities will come flooding and bouncing into your life. With blessings of health,

Patricia Bragg

RECOMMENDED BLOOD CHEMISTRY VALUES

- Total Cholesterol:
  180 mg/dl or less,
  150 mg/dl or less (optimal)
- HDL cholesterol:
  Men: 46 mg/dl or more,
  Women: 56 mg/dl or more
  Ages 2-12: 120-140 mg/dl

- HDL Cholesterol Ratio 3.2 or less
- LDL Cholesterol: 120 or less
- Glucose 50-100 md/dl

PURE WATER — ESSENTIAL FOR HEALTH!

Distilled water is one of the world's best and purest waters! It is excellent for detoxification and fasting programs and for helping clean out all the cells, organs, and fluids of the body because it can help carry away so many harmful substances!

Water from chemically-treated public water systems and even from many wells and springs is likely to be loaded with poisonous chemicals and toxic trace elements.

Depending upon the kind of piping that the water has been run through, the water in our homes, offices, schools, hospitals, etc., is likely to be overloaded with zinc (from old-fashioned galvanized pipes) or with copper and cadmium (from copper pipes). These trace elements are released in excessive quantity by the chemical action of the water on the metals of the water pipes.

Yes, pure water is essential for health, either from the natural juices of vegetables, fruits, and other foods, or from the water of high purity obtained by steam distillation which is the best method, or by one of the new high-efficiency deionization processes.

The body is constantly working for you . . . breaking down old bone and tissue cells and replacing them with new ones. As the body casts off the old minerals and other products of broken-down cells, it must obtain new supplies of the essential elements for the new cells. Moreover, Scientists are only now beginning to understand that various kinds of dental problems, different types of arthritis, and even some forms of hardening of the arteries are due to varying kinds of imbalances in the levels of calcium, phosphorus, and magnesium in the body. Disorders can also be caused by imbalances in the ratios of various minerals to each other.

Each individual healthy body requires a proper balance within itself of all the nutritive elements. It is just as bad for any individual to have too much of one item as it is to have too little of that one or of another one. It takes appropriate levels of phosphorus and magnesium to keep calcium in solution so it can be formed into new cells of bone and teeth. Yet, there must not be too much of those nor too little calcium in the diet, or old bone will be taken away but new bone will not be formed.

In addition, we now know that diets which are unbalanced and inappropriate for a given individual can deplete the body of calcium, magnesium, potassium, and other major and minor elements.

Diets which are high in meats, fish, eggs, grains, nuts, seeds, or their products may provide unbalanced excesses of phosphorus which will deplete calcium and magnesium from the bones and tissues of the body and cause them to be lost in the urine.

A diet high in fats will tend to increase the uptake of phosphorus from the intestines relative to calcium and other basic minerals. Such a high-fat diet can produce losses of calcium, magnesium, and other basic minerals in the same way a high-phosphorus diet does.

Diets excessively high in fruits or their juices may provide unbalanced excesses of potassium in the body, and calcium and magnesium will again be lost from the body through the urine.

Deficiencies of calcium and magnesium . . . for example can produce all kinds of problems in the body ranging from dental decay and osteoporosis to muscular cramping, hyper-activity, muscular twitching, poor sleep patterns, and excessive frequency of uncontrolled patterns of urination. Similarly, deficiencies of other minerals, or imbalances in the levels of those minerals, can produce many other problems in the body.

Therefore, it is important to clean and detoxify the body through fasting and through using distilled or other pure water as well as healthy organically-grown vegetable and fruit juices. At the same time, it is also important to provide the body with adequate sources of new minerals. This can be done by eating a widely-distributed diet of wholesome vegetables, including kelp and other sea vegetables for adults and healthy mother's milk for infants, and certified raw goat's or cow's milk for those children and adults who are not adversely affected by milk products . . . but most processed home homogenized milks we do not suggest using.

But, despite dietary sources such as these, many adults and children in so-called civilized cultures will be found to have low levels of essential minerals in their bodies due to losses caused by coffee, tea, carbonated beverages, and long-term bad diets containing too much sugar and other sweets as well as products made from refined flours and containing refined table salt.

In addition, the body's organ systems can be thrown out of balance by continuing stress, by toxins in our air and water, by disease-produced injuries, and by pre-natal deficiencies in the mother's diet or life style.

As a result, many, if not most people in our so-called civilization may need to take mineral supplements such as the new chelated multiple mineral preparations as well as a broad-range multiple-vitamin tablet.

BORON – MIRACLE TRACE MINERAL FOR HEALTHY BONES

BORON – Trace mineral for healthy bones helps the body have more Calcium, Mineral & Hormones! Boron is found in vegetables, fruits, nut and especially good sources are broccoli, prunes, dates, raisins, almonds, peanuts and soybeans.

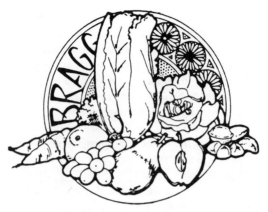

FROM THE AUTHORS

This book was written for YOU. It can be your passport to the Good Life. We Professional Nutritionists join hands in one common objective — a high standard of health for all and many added years to your life. Scientific Nutrition points the way — Nature's Way — the only lasting way to build a body free of degenerative diseases and premature aging. This book teaches you how to work with Nature and not against her. Doctors, dentists, and others who care for the sick, try to repair depleted tissues which too often mend poorly if at all. Many of them praise the spreading of this new scientific message of natural foods and methods for long-lasting health and youthfulness at any age. To speed the spreading of this tremendous message, this book was written.

Statements in this book are recitals of scientific findings, known facts of physiology, biological therapeutics, and reference to ancient writings as they are found. Paul C. Bragg has been practicing the natural methods of living for over 70 years, with highly beneficial results, knowing they are safe and of great value to others, and his daughter Patricia Bragg works with him to carry on the Health Crusade. They make no claims as to what the methods cited in this book will do for one in any given situation, and assume no obligation because of opinions expressed.

No cure for disease is offered in this book. No foods or diets are offered for the treatment or cure of any specific ailment. Nor is it intended as, or to be used as, literature for any food product. Paul C. Bragg and Patricia Bragg express their opinions solely as Public Health Educators, Professional Nutritionists and Teachers.

Certain persons considered experts may disagree with one or more statements in this book, as the same relate to various nutritional recommendations. However, any such statements are considered, nevertheless, to be factual, as based upon long-time experience of Paul C. Bragg and Patricia Bragg in the field of human health.

SEND FOR IMPORTANT
FREE
HEALTH BULLETINS

Let Patricia Bragg send you, your relatives and friends the latest
News Bulletins on Health and Nutrition Discoveries. These are
sent periodically. Please enclose two stamps for each U.S.A.
name listed. Foreign listings send international postal reply
coupons. Please print or type addresses, thank you.

HEALTH SCIENCE Box 7, Santa Barbara, California 93102 U.S.A.

●
_____
Name

_____ ( ) _____
Address   Phone

_____
City   State   Zip Code

●
_____
Name

_____ ( ) _____
Address   Phone

_____
City   State   Zip Code

●
_____
Name

_____ ( ) _____
Address   Phone

_____
City   State   Zip Code

●
_____
Name

_____ ( ) _____
Address   Phone

_____
City   State   Zip Code

●
_____
Name

_____ ( ) _____
Address   Phone

_____
City   State   Zip Code

BRAGG ALL NATURAL LIQUID AMINOS
Order Form

Delicious, Healthy Alternative to Tamari-Soy Sauce

BRAGG LIQUID AMINOS — Nutrition you need...taste you will love...a family favorite for over 75 years. A delicious source of nutritious life-renewing protein from soybeans only. Add to or spray over casseroles, soups, sauces, gravies, potatoes, popcorn, and vegetables. An ideal "pick-me-up" broth at work, home or the gym. Gourmet health replacement for Tamari & Soy Sauce. Start today and add more Amino Acids for healthy living to your daily diet — the easy BRAGG LIQUID AMINOS Way!

DASH or SPRAY for NEW TASTE DELIGHTS! PROVEN & ENJOYED BY MILLIONS.

DELICIOUS, NUTRITIOUS, FAMILY FAVORITE FOR OVER 75 YEARS!

Dash of Bragg Aminos Brings New Taste Delights to Season:
- Salads
- Dressings
- Soups
- Vegies
- Rice/Beans
- Tofu
- Tempeh
- Wok foods
- Stir-frys
- Casseroles & Potatoes
- Meats
- Poultry
- Fish
- Popcorn
- Gravies
- Sauces
- Macrobiotics

Pure Soybeans and Pure Water Only
- No Added Sodium
- No Coloring Agents
- No Preservatives
- Not Fermented
- No Chemicals
- No Additives
- No MSG

BRAGG LIQUID AMINOS

SIZE	PRICE	SHIPPING	AMT.	TOTAL $
16 oz.	$ 3.95 ea.	Please add $3.00 for 1st bottle/$1.50 for each additional bottle		.
32 oz.	$ 6.45 ea.	Please add $3.90 for 1st bottle/$1.90 for each additional bottle		.
16 oz.	$ 47.40 ea.	Case/12 bottles add $9.00 per case		.
32 oz.	$ 77.40 ea.	Case/12 bottles add $14.00 per case		.

Total Aminos	$	.
Shipping & Handling		.
Total Enclosed	$	.

Please Specify: (U.S. Funds Only)

☐ Check ☐ Money Order ☐ Cash ☐ Credit Card

Charge My Order To: ☐ Visa ☐ MasterCard

Credit Card Number: _ _ _ _ — _ _ _ _ — _ _ _ _ — _ _ _ _   Card Expires: Month | Year

MasterCard VISA Signature:_____

CREDIT CARD CUSTOMERS ONLY USE OUR FAST PHONE SERVICE: (800) 446-1990

In a hurry? Call **(805) 968-1028**. We can accept MasterCard & VISA phone orders only. Please prepare your order using this order form. It will speed your call & serve as your order record. Hours: 9 to 4 pm Pacific Time, Monday to Thursday ... or you can fax your order to: **FAX (805) 968-1001**.

Mail to: **HEALTH SCIENCE, Box 7, Santa Barbara, CA 93102 USA**

Please Print or Type — Be sure to give street & house number to facilitate delivery

A-BOF-9201

Name _____

Address _____ Apt. No. _____

City _____ State _____

( ) _____
Phone   Zip _ _ _ _ _

Bragg Aminos —Taste You Love, Nutrition You Need

SEND FOR IMPORTANT
FREE
HEALTH BULLETINS

Let Patricia Bragg send you, your relatives and friends the latest News Bulletins on Health and Nutrition Discoveries. These are sent periodically. Please enclose two stamps for each U.S.A. name listed. Foreign listings send international postal reply coupons. Please print or type addresses, thank you.

HEALTH SCIENCE Box 7, Santa Barbara, California 93102 U.S.A.

●
_____
Name

_____ ( ) _____
Address   Phone

_____
City   State   Zip Code

●
_____
Name

_____ ( ) _____
Address   Phone

_____
City   State   Zip Code

●
_____
Name

_____ ( ) _____
Address   Phone

_____
City   State   Zip Code

●
_____
Name

_____ ( ) _____
Address   Phone

_____
City   State   Zip Code

●
_____
Name

_____ ( ) _____
Address   Phone

_____
City   State   Zip Code

PAUL C. BRAGG N.D., Ph.D.

Life Extension Specialist • World Health Crusader
Lecturer and Advisor to Olympic Athletes, Royalty, and Stars
Originator of Health Food Stores - Now World-wide

For almost a Century, Living Proof that his
"Health and Fitness Way of Life" Works Wonders!

Paul C. Bragg is the Father of the Health Movement in America. This dynamic Crusader for worldwide health and fitness is responsible for more "firsts" in the history of Health than any other individual. Here are a few of his incredible pioneering achievements that the world now enjoys:

- Bragg originated, named and opened the first "Health Food Store" in America.
- Bragg Crusades pioneered the first Health Lectures across America, inspiring followers to open health stores in cities across the land and now world-wide.
- Bragg introduced pineapple juice and tomato juice to the American public.
- He was the first to introduce and distribute honey nationwide.
- He introduced Juice Therapy in America by importing the first hand-juicers.
- Bragg pioneered Radio Health Programs from Hollywood three times daily. Paul and Patricia pioneered a Health TV show from Hollywood to spread "Health and Happiness"... the name of the show! It included exercises, health recipes, visual demonstrations, and guest appearances of famous, health-minded people.
- He created the first health foods & products and made them available nation-wide: herb teas, health beverages, seven-grain cereals and crackers, health cosmetics, health candies, vitamins and mineral supplements, wheat germ, digestive enzymes from papaya, herbs & kelp seasonings, amino acids from soybeans. He inspired others to follow and now thousands of health items are available worldwide.
- He opened the first health restaurants and health spas in America.

Crippled by TB as a teenager, Bragg developed his own eating, breathing and exercising program to rebuild his body into an ageless, tireless, painfree citadel of glowing, radiant health. He excelled in running, swimming, biking, progressive weight training, and mountain-climbing. He made an early pledge to God, in return for his renewed health, to spend the rest of his life showing others the road to health... Paul Bragg made good his pledge!

A living legend and beloved counselor to millions, Bragg was the inspiration and personal advisor on diet and fitness to top Olympic Stars from 4-time swimming Gold Medalist Murray Rose to 3-time track Gold Medalist Betty Cuthbert of Australia, his relative Don Bragg (pole-vaulting Gold Medalist), and countless others. Jack LaLanne, "the original TV King of Fitness," says, "Bragg saved my life at age 15 when I attended the Bragg Crusade in Oakland, California." From the earliest days, Bragg was advisor to the greatest Hollywood Stars, and to giants of American Business. J. C. Penney, Del E. Webb, and Conrad Hilton are just a few that he inspired to long, successful, healthy, active lives!

Dr. Bragg changed the lives of millions worldwide in all walks of life... through his Health Crusades, Books, Tapes and Radio, TV and personal appearances.

HEALTH SCIENCE Box 7, Santa Barbara, California 93102 U.S.A.

PATRICIA BRAGG N.D., Ph.D.
Angel of Health
Lecturer, Author, Nutritionist, Health Educator & Fitness Advisor to World Leaders, Glamorous Hollywood Stars, Singers, Dancers & Athletes.

Daughter of the world renowned health authority, Paul C. Bragg, Patricia Bragg has won international fame on her own in this field. She conducts Health and Fitness Seminars for Women's, Men's, Youth and Church Groups throughout the world... and promotes Bragg "How-To, Self-Health" Books in Lectures, on Radio and Television Talk Shows throughout the English-speaking world. Consultants to Presidents and Royalty, to the Stars of Stage, Screen and TV and to Champion Athletes, Patricia Bragg and her father are Co-Authors of the Bragg Health Library of Instructive, Inspiring Books that promote a healthy lifestyle for a long, vital, active life!

Patricia herself is the symbol of perpetual youth and super energy. She is a living and sparkling example of hers and her father's healthy lifestyle precepts and this she shares world-wide.

A fifth generation Californian on her mother's side, Patricia was reared by the Natural Health Method from infancy. In school, she not only excelled in athletics but also won high honors in her studies and her counseling. She is an accomplished musician and dancer... as well as tennis player, swimmer and mountain climber... and the youngest woman ever to be granted a U.S. Patent. Patricia is a popular gifted Health Teacher and a dynamic, in-demand Talk Show Guest where she spreads simple, easy-to-follow health teachings for everyone.

Man's body is the Temple of the Holy Spirit, and our creator wants us filled with Joy and Health for a long walk with Him for Eternity. The Bragg Crusade of Health and Fitness (3 John 2) has carried her around the world... spreading physical, spiritual, emotional and mental health and joy. Health is our birthright and Patricia teaches how to prevent the destruction of our health from man-made wrong habits of living.

Patricia's been Health Consultant to American Presidents and to the British Royal Family, to Betty Cuthbert, Australia's "Golden Girl" who holds 16 world records and four Olympic gold medals in women's track and to New Zealand's Olympic Track Star Allison Roe. Among those who come to her for advice are some of Hollywood's top starts from Clint Eastwood to the ever youthful singing group The Beach Boys and their families, singing stars of the Metropolitan Opera and top ballet stars. Patricia's message is of world-wide appeal to the people of all ages, nationalities and walks-of-life. Those who follow the Bragg Health Books and attend the Crusades are living testimonials like Jack LaLanne proved.

Patricia gives "Bragg Super Healthy Lifestyle Living" Seminars and Lectures world-wide. These are life-changing and millions have benefited with a longer, healthier life, and she would love to share with your clubs, groups, corps., churches, etc. Also, she is a perfect radio and T.V. talk show guest to spread the message of health and fitness in your area. Write or call for requests and information:

HEALTH SCIENCE, BOX 7, SANTA BARBARA, CA 93102 1-805-968-1028